Dermo
Neuro
Modulating

MANUAL TREATMENT FOR
PERIPHERAL NERVES AND
ESPECIALLY CUTANEOUS NERVES

Diane Jacobs

foreword by *JASON SILVERNAIL PT*

DermoNeuroModulating

Copyright © 2016 by Diane Jacobs

No part of this publication may be reproduced, distributed, or transmitted in any form or by any means, including photocopying, recording, or other electronic or mechanical methods, without the prior written permission of the author, except in the case of brief quotations embodied in critical reviews and certain other non-commercial uses permitted by copyright law.

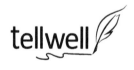

Tellwell Talent

www.tellwell.ca

ISBN

978-1-987985-19-1 (Hardcover)

978-1-987985-18-4 (Paperback)

978-1-987985-20-7 (eBook)

Contents

Foreword

It's a great pleasure to introduce you to this wonderful book. In the busy world of medicine, in a crowded field of systems, approaches, copyrighted tools and techniques in physical medicine and rehabilitation, Diane Jacobs developed Dermoneuromodulating, or DNM. In the constantly-shifting landscape of the marketing of medicine, she built this approach from the ground up to be the opposite of the kind of slickly-marketed, money-focused commodity that we so often see. It turns out that the things that make DNM so different and so valuable are the some of the same things that make Diane so different and so valued by her professional colleagues and friends.

Diane is an autodidact, and this makes DNM accessible. Realizing some time ago that you didn't need a PhD to research and read and understand things you cared about, she taught herself neuroscience and pain mechanisms at a time when the field was rapidly evolving (in truth, it still is). She remains one of the most-informed and well-read people that I know on these topics. She did this work so she could bring this form of treatment to as many people as possible – not just medical practitioners such as physical therapists and physicians, but massage therapists, chiropractors, Rolfers, Feldenkrais practitioners, anyone who could use a hands-on approach to help others. Diane knows more about touch sensation, perception, and pain neuroscience than almost anyone else I know - and I know a lot of researchers in these areas. She learned it all the old-fashioned way - by reading, thinking, and making connections between things the way no one else has.

Diane is humble, so DNM doesn't make lofty claims of success with a flashy marketing campaign. In fact, you might find the understated tone of the manual a nice contrast with the over-the-top approaches of other systems. No miracle stories, no multiple levels of certification, no saving of the good material for 'the advanced course', just a consistent set of principles based on the science, her experience in manual therapy, and an honest attempt to meld the two responsibly and treat patients gently.

Diane cares about making her practice defensible with science, so DNM's mechanistic explanations are entirely consistent with neuroscience. Diane Jacobs is the anti-guru. I have seen her present her ideas publicly in online forums for the last 12 years, taking criticism from anyone to test her assumptions, review her knowledge of the relevant basic science, and expose any reasoning errors she may have made. She has accepted critical feedback from world-famous neuroscientists as well as anonymous forum participants. She's been wrong sometimes, right most of the time, and almost always gracious and thoughtful in her interactions. I have seen her accept corrections on her reasoning from experts with humility and grace. I've also seen her take the time to explain herself to the most unreasonable forum troll – she's changed many minds over the years with her persistence and her willingness to think out loud and subject her ideas to scrutiny.

She accepted early teaching opportunities with reluctance, initially requiring several rounds of encouragement behind the closed doors of the SomaSimple web forum's moderator section. I think at first she honestly couldn't see why people would want to hear her speak. She wasn't a famous researcher with a PhD, she hadn't published randomized trials, she wasn't advertising her course on the pages of therapy journals. But it's for all those reasons that we wanted to hear her. When we saw Diane stand up and speak, I think many of us saw a little of ourselves. We saw an earnest and caring clinician trying to pull together a defensible practice of care with low-cost, low-risk, noninvasive care. Without fancy gadgets, expensive tools, or thousand-dollar certifications. With just two hands, a grasp of the science, a commitment to gentle treatment, and an honest, unpretentious caring for patients. If that kind of practice appeals to you, I think you'll like what you find here. I hope you also appreciate what Diane has poured 15 years of effort and time into and spent countless hours of reading to build for all of us. What a true gift you are about to open. Hurry up and get to it.

Jason Silvernail DPT, DSc, FAAOMPT
Northern Virginia, USA
2016

Preface

I would like to acknowledge all those who supported this effort, especially Bas Asselbergs for edits, Bruce Schonfeld for advice on structure, Jason Silvernail for his gracious foreword, and Sandy Hilton for her bluntness as we conversed over a glass of wine at the 2016 San Diego Pain Summit, "Diane, 85% done is good enough. Send it in."

I thank the anatomy lab at U.B.C. for allowing a non-academic access to dissect cutaneous rami in 2007. I thank Loren Rex, D.O., who taught manual therapy at the URSA foundation in Edmonds, Wa., (where I spent way too many weekends throughout the 1990's and no small amount of money, searching for answers that I finally had to carefully cobble together for myself). I thank those PTs who gained my rapt attention by bringing a wave of pain science into physical and manual therapy - David Butler, Louis Gifford, Michael Shacklock, Lorimer Moseley, and those who came before them. Here in Canada, thank you to Angela Busch at U. Sask. who helped design a study to test DNM in 2006. Thank you to Dave Walton, Neil Pearson, Debbie Patterson, Mike Sangster, and Lesley Singer, who took the little idea Nick Matheson had hatched in 2004, and that I had carried forward through to 2005, and developed the Canadian Physiotherapy Pain Science Division, finally approved by CPA in 2009. Thank you to Bahram Jam in Toronto and Donald Soule in Chicago who helped clarify images and concepts that appear in the book. Thank you to practitioners all over the world who have already embraced and are teaching DNM to others in their respective countries in their respective languages, people like Rey Allen, Rajam Roose, Jason Erickson, Julie Porter, Jeff Rockwell, Erik Ouellet, Michael Reoch, Louise Tremblay. Together, we can make manual therapy into something that makes more sense while being kinder and less uncomfortable for people who are already in pain.

I doubt this book would ever have emerged at all, had it not been for Bernard Delalande in France who developed SomaSimple in 2004, where for a number of years I lived every day for hours, found a writing voice and learned how to use it. Most of my virtual discussion companions still moderate there – Jason and Bas, Barrett Dorko, Cory Blickenstaff, John Ware, Kory Zimney,

Rod Hendrickson, Carol Lynn Chevrier and many others. Despite bumps along the way, I think we have come to understand and respect each other quite well.

I dedicate this effort to Jon Newman, another SomaSimple moderator who I am so grateful to have met in person in 2005; he helped me with the first draft way back in 2007 and passed away much too young in 2012.

Diane Jacobs PT
Weyburn, Saskatchewan, Canada

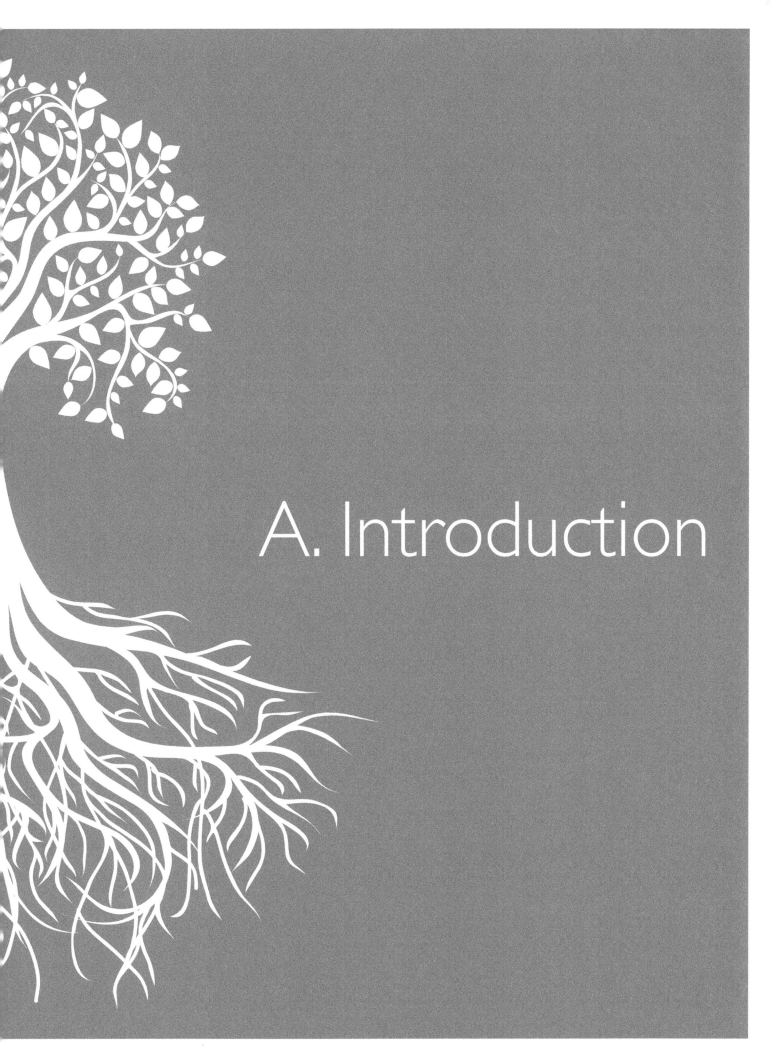

A. Introduction

A Fresh Look At Manual Therapy

What would happen if manual therapists were to focus on brain function, spinal cord function, and nerve function, instead of tissue?

I think manual therapy would become kinder. I think we would listen very closely to patients' accounts of their pain, explain nerves in detail, explain pain much better in ways patients could understand, with their own story details woven back in. I think we would insist that our patients own and exercise locus of control over treatment, in particular regarding their own comfort levels. I think any results from manual therapy provided, and any results from it and from any movement homework afterward, would be considered by both parties, and both parties' brains, as having been arrived at mutually, interactively. I think we therapists would enhance our abilities to elicit favourable descending modulation for pain from another's brain, through awareness of how touch and handling of peripheral nerve is perceived by the brain attached, instead of performing futile attempts to change structure or tissue.

This manual is my fantasy of how such manual therapy could be conceptualized and carried out by manual practitioners of any kind. It is deliberately visual because most people learn easier with pictures. The pictures show my ideas on how to move nerves. It contains suggestions for treatment of specific nerves; the treatment approaches, however, are by no means specific. The manual is not encyclopedic; practitioners are completely free to make up new treatment approaches or use old ones to new purpose.

The objectives are simple:

1. to help keep manual therapy alive
2. to make it more congruent with pain science and neuroscience
3. to help more patients be treated more kindly
4. to help manual therapy practitioners understand the nervous system better and provide manual therapy from that standpoint.

Usually in books like this the front chapters lay out all the reasoning and the treatment section is at the back. I have laid this book out in reverse order; the treatment ideas are in front, followed by a visual appendix of each nerve root and what it innervates. At the back are referenced chapters that include background for each of the following premises.

PREMISES

As a physical therapist for 45 years, 3 decades of which I have primarily been a manual therapist, and through the past 15 years of studying pain science, I have accepted the following ideas:

1. **Pain is in the nervous system**. There are all sorts of definitions for pain, but let us stick with the official one from the International Association for the Study of Pain (IASP):

   "An unpleasant sensory and emotional experience associated with actual or potential tissue damage, or described in terms of such damage." - http://www.iasp-pain.org/Taxonomy#Pain

   The word "potential" in this definition suggests to us that pain is not irrevocably correlated to tissue damage, only to the brain's own opinion about the state of its body. When we experience pain, it is *we* for whom the experience is unpleasant, sensory, and emotional. Our brains do not particularly care what "we" experience, which might be "pain"; they just do their own work, filtering input, in the moment, from a large number of sources, including whatever experiences we have had through a lifetime, the current context they are in, and ongoing sensory input, to decide what current reality is. Our spinal cords do not care; their job is to reflexively protect and guard. If you touch a hot surface like the burner of a stove, by accident, your spinal cord will detect "danger" and have pulled your hand off faster than the nociceptive information has even reached your brain to be processed as "painful," or not. To sum up, pain is not an input from structural tissue, as is frequently implied.

2. **The brain is predictive, not reactive**. This means it takes account of everything, then ignores most of it. It exhibits hierarchical functions, which means it is great at ignoring and inhibiting sensory input and feedback it regards as inconsequential. It exhibits parallel functions, which means that its representational maps interlink and interact with each other both forward and backward within the sensory stream. It uses feature extraction when triggered by a stimulus, which means that ever more specific features of the sensory world are 'extracted' as sensory info flows forward through the brain, and these will be the features *important to the creature sensing them* - in our case, human creatures.

a.   This means, to a large extent we can influence our patients into paying attention to whatever we *think* (as therapists) they should pay attention to during treatment and between treatments.

b.   This is a *professional responsibility*: we owe it to our patients to not distract them with meaningless observations or concepts, which could be harmful by being noceboic. We owe them the service of helping them to come into improved relationship with their own nervous systems, of which they are only the conscious, self-aware social-seeking part, tip of an iceberg.

3.   **The brain has evolved to filter out nociceptive information**. And it usually does, easily, except for when biologically reactive, physiological positive feedback loops emerge that *amplify* nociceptive input, enhance, and maintain it, or when an individual has become stressed to the point that their brain's endogenous opioid production may have become impaired.

4.   **We treat pain problems, not tissue**. Pain might be felt as strictly physical. It might start out perceived as physical and become emotionally overlain. It may start out as a small problem that turns into something a lot bigger. It is usually a mixed bag. Sometimes it will be injury-related; pain that lasts far longer than it is useful, long past a time frame in which healing should be complete, can be baffling and distressing. Often it can come seemingly out of nowhere. Intense pain that seems to have come out of nowhere can be bewildering, shocking, as well as distressing. There will always be people who must deal with some pain problem. Our job is to help them with that, if they ask us to, to recognize kinds of pain we cannot help, and refer out if necessary – not offer false hope.

5.   **We treat pain, not medical conditions**. If we try to claim we can treat medical *conditions* with manual therapy, in my opinion we exceed our scopes of practice. We may be able to help people alleviate some of the *pain* that may be associated with them, however, even if just temporarily.

We can help a lot with *non*-medical pain, i.e., pain in which medical red flags have been ruled out. The most common kind that manual therapy may help is pain

·   of any duration

·   no recent tissue disruption (e.g., fracture)

·   usually confined to a neuroanatomically plausible region

·   often associated with having not moved enough or having moved too much

In short, we are pretty good at treating "mechanical" pain, i.e., pain that changes with position or use or movement, and is usually accompanied by secondary hyperalgesia (tenderness or "sore spots"). See tunnel syndromes and "neuritis" later in the book for more about this kind of pain phenomenon.

There are some chronic pain "syndromes" for which manual therapy is of little or no value, e.g., fibromyalgia, or could even make worse, e.g. "wind-up" pain. Lucky for us, people with wind-up pain, or hyperpathia, are rare. But be careful. Take a really good history. There are some people with pain we simply should not try to treat using manual therapy.

6. **We cannot actually "touch" anything, except skin.** This seems obvious, but way too many manual therapy treatment systems *still* try to target bones or muscle lying deep beneath the *surface* layer, a thick rubbery, mobile layer of highly innervated, physiologically important, force-dissipating, slidey, frictionless skin organ, ignoring said skin organ and all the nerves embedded within it in the process.

   The receptive fields of many kinds of sensory neurons overlap at the surface: just touching skin in a properly prepared patient will send a cascade of novel sensory information through to the brain and to all its maps. We need to respect the skin organ, think about it, and learn how to work with it, instead of against it.

7. **The nervous system is needy, greedy, and sensitive.** All the neurons in the whole body and brain comprise only about 2% of the whole body, but use 25% of all available oxygen and glucose, 24/7. They can only get what they need through adequate blood supply. There are 72 kilometers or 45 miles of peripheral nerve in a human body. Nerves are long, walled cylinders that protect neurons. Getting blood through small thin regional vessels into and out of nerve is somewhat perilous, as vascular structures may be pulled in different directions than the nerves they supply. If a nerve does not receive adequate blood supply, because of mechanical tension affecting regional vessels feeding it, or it becomes backed up from mechanical tension affecting regional vessels that drain it, its own nociceptive innervation can activate.

8. **Tunnel syndromes:** A tunnel syndrome is basically a cranky nerve whose tunnel has become a compressive or tensional threat to the neurons inside it; nociceptive neurons embedded within the nerve walls that confine them signal "danger." Causes can be medical or metabolic or hormonal (e.g., pregnancy, diabetes, myxedema), or non-medical. Non-medical tunnel syndromes may arise because of too much movement of a repetitive kind, or simply not enough movement of any kind. (Couch potatoes, look out.) Nociceptive neurons within a nerve, complaining, activate others nearby, to create a so-called sterile inflammation, or peripheral sensitization, inside the nerve itself. "Neuritis" is currently classified by IASP as a special category of neuropathic pain. This is a kind of persisting pain that manual therapy can be very useful for treating.

9. **Motion is lotion.** There are 72 km or 45 miles of peripheral nerve in a human body. Moving nerves therapeutically and strategically helps to maintain their physiological and biological health. Healthy nerves that are well fed and drained through adequate and varied movement, do not contribute to pain experiences. Sometimes however, because of many reasons which may

involve pathological processes, or through injury long ago, too much of one kind of movement, or not enough variation of movement, nerves can develop tunnel syndromes. People can easily be taught how to look after their own nerves, once they understand ways in which they may be unconsciously contributing to the problem.

10. **Social grooming**. Sometimes movement by itself is not enough to change a pain experience, once it has established itself. That is where we manual therapists fit in. We can provide first aid to the person, to their nervous system, and their nerves.

We can help people relieve their stress, especially the stress of having pain, by:

- providing a safe context for them
- listening carefully to them,
- explaining pain to them
- explaining to them that moving their nerves with our hands may help a lot without hurting them more, and
- teaching them how to move their own nerves.
- We can help brains, and nervous systems as a whole, by:
- providing innocuous sensory input into them
- not overwhelming their threat-detective mechanisms
- giving them space, and time, to change their predictive mechanisms, and pain and motor output
- helping them inhibit spinal cord protective mechanisms with descending modulation

We can provide first aid to nerves by moving them as specifically as we can.

11. **Less is more:** Examine your manual therapy assumptions, constantly. Provide patients with favourable context and plenty of pain education; treat them slowly, thoughtfully, and carefully. This, more than anything, will help your manual efforts to be effective. Keep your hands clean, warm, slow, light, kind, responsive, intelligent. Make sure they understand they are in charge of the handling, and can interrupt it at the slightest discomfort. Above all, do no harm.

WHY BRING A NEW NAME INTO MANUAL THERAPY?

"Dermo" means skin. "Neuro" means nerve. "Modulating" or "-ion" means change. The name has been registered with Creative Commons. This means, I do not "own" it and cannot trademark it, nor can anyone else "own" it or trademark it; it is a public domain name that anyone who wants to consider nervous system rather than structural tissue when they treat can use if they wish.

Any lasting change that occurs within the patient and their body is the result of a patient' brain having decided to change its own output, not because a manual therapist has any special, e:

pensively obtained manual skill set, or magical power in their hands. Any manual approach by any name that succeeds in reducing pain, will inherently be dermoneuromodulatory, regardless of what the practitioner may "think" they are doing, biomechanically or what have you: physical treatment is interactive between two conscious, awake, aware human nervous systems, not operative by one. DNM is therefore an explanatory model for any kind of slow, careful manual therapy, more than it is a treatment model.

The overall goal of DNM treatment is to reduce movement-restricting pain felt by the patient as though it is coming from the body. The only *physical* target is nerve and nerve physiology.

All approaches included this book are "neurodynamic": this means, directed toward the simple objective of moving nerves, giving them more room to slide, unloading them rather than loading them more, helping them feed and drain. Approaches can be easily combined.

Where is the evidence?

Although colleagues and I conducted a pilot study using a DNM approach, it remains unpublished; statistical analysis of the results revealed, disappointingly, that data booklets had been backfilled by study participants.

Perhaps in the future better research designs will ensue. I decided to publish this manual anyway.

Skin stretch approach (the "dermo" of dermoneuromodulating)

Special attention is given to cutaneous nerves in this treatment model. Why? Because they have been largely overlooked in other treatment systems and models, both as a source of pain and as a treatment target. Every cubic centimeter of skin organ has a nerve or portion thereof, supplying it, embedded into it. It is easy to move skin relative to the rest of the body.

Cutaneous nerves rise up out of the depths of the body, surface through dense body wall into the skin organ, and run parallel to it, behind or within it. Sore spots on the surface of the body coincide to a large extent with the "grommet holes" or exit points for these nerves that emerge from beneath and into the skin organ. If you learn the main locations for these, you can teach yourself to drag skin *away* from them, which will move the nerve out of them a little farther. Think of ice fishing – pulling a line up and out through a hole in the ice. This seems to work best if you follow the path the nerve is going already. But be ready to be creative – not all nerves in people are like the ones in the anatomy books. They do all sorts of creative anastomosing, which means a nerve physically joins into a different nerve beside it. Some people are missing entire nerves, and some other nerve does the job of the missing nerve. You have to embrace uncertainty, because you simply cannot know what another person's detailed neural anatomy really is.

Multiple rami branch off these nerves within the skin organ, which is actually quite thick, and travel to its surface inside tubular skin ligaments. These ligaments provide directional preference – if you try to move skin against them, you will feel resistance.

It is a good idea to position people comfortably. I use sidelying most of the time, so that the arms and legs can be folded to rest on pillows, which takes tension out of the entire peripheral nervous system. Our peripheral nervous system evolved in quadrupeds (most of it, anyway), so it seems reasonable that allowing it to adopt some sort of quadruped position whenever possible will help the entire peripheral neural tree become more slack and comfortable.

Now, get out your inquisitive fingers, because palpatory skill does have a role to play: cranky nerves feel harder, thicker, and wirier than they should.

Sometimes a good-sized three-dimensional zone within someone's skin organ will feel swollen and turgid, as if it were a "thing." In this treatment system, such palpable hardness is considered to be merely abnormal autonomic motor output within a small anatomic compartment.

I refer to these fleeting anomalies as "blumps," a place marker term that carries no conceptual baggage needing to be deconstructed. Perhaps fluid has become backed up into a compartment and has not been able to escape, due to a minor positive feedback loop, possibly, or some prolonged position or lack of overall movement by the person. It does not matter in the end: such "blumps" go away easily with treatment. So, with full embrace of post hoc ergo propter hoc reasoning, I presume they *must therefore have been due* merely to a small neural entrapment that was close enough to the surface that one could feel them with one's fingers.

We all have these: nimble, searching fingers, replete with tiny receptive fields, massive sensory-discriminative capacity, and an astonishingly large portion of the real estate devoted to processing information from them in the representational map in one's own human somatosensory cortex, about a third of that available for decoding information from one's entire body surface. Use the heck out of your inquisitive fingers. If people can learn how to read Braille with their fingertips, people can learn to find "blumps," which are a lot bigger. We can use our time, and our ability to be still and patient, to figure out how to help them disappear, without hurting patients in the process.

It is helpful to us practitioners, who are like pilots flying through the fog of uncertainty, to have a relationship with the person inside the nervous system we are trying to help. They can help guide us, once we teach them how. When our fingers find tissue that does not feel homogeneous, that feels like a "blump," we can ask the individual we are treating if it feels tender to them. Tenderness represents secondary hyperalgesia. If it does feel tender, then we have gained another clue to the puzzle, and another node of connection to our patient. We have already assured them we are not going to hurt them, but that we need to check to make sure we are addressing something that is connected to their nervous system; then we proceed to *un*load it, *de*compress it (not squash it or stick needles into it). By dragging skin gently away *from* it, it will soften and become less tender. Sometimes it will soften immediately but take a bit longer to become non-tender. Sometimes the tenderness vanishes immediately, and it will take a longer while to soften. You never know. In any case, your job is to stay there with it, keep it unloaded, until the patient's nervous system has had enough time to change itself and its autonomic motor output. Sometimes this takes two minutes. Sometimes it takes 10 minutes. A lot of times, treatment involving passive movement of skin will seem like watching paint dry. Think of it as a good opportunity to learn patience and stillness and silence.

The people being treated do not seem to mind. They usually go off into a quiet state in which they are half dreaming, perhaps feeling all the opioids swishing through the representational maps in their brains, perhaps also in their bodies, giving long sighs, relaxing into gravity as their patterns of tension give way at the spinal cord level, as reflexive withdrawal action mediated by their spinal cord succumbs to descending inhibition. Sometimes people's bodies will clunk loudly, spontaneously. This always makes me smile. No need to go learn expensive ways to forcibly manipulate people dangerously at high velocities – such an impatient thing to do - let nature do all that work for you instead. Let nervous systems figure out how to do all their own heavy lifting, self-correction, positive feedback loop dismantling. I see my task as akin to holding up a kinaesthetic flashlight so that a brain can see a pain problem well enough to realize it represents a waste of its energy and talents, and devise a solution that best suits it.

When it feels as though nothing more is happening under your fingers, you can gently restore the skin to its normal position, and move on. I am a test-retest sort of person, so I will usually ask the patient to stand up and try the movement again, the movement they were having trouble doing, the one they could not do without pain, to see if it works better now. If they can, this is yet more post hoc confirmation that I may just have been able to affect their brain through the large, stretch-receptive neuronal end organs right inside their skin organ – the ones attached to thickly myelinated fast fibres that extend without stopping all the way from the surface of their skin, up the fast dorsal columns of the spinal cord straight up to dorsal column nuclei in the medulla, so fast they can outrace any information plodding in along thin unmyelinated neurons with all those synapses in the dorsal horn, where their information can be stalled or ignored by descending modulation.

If we *can* get non-noxious information into a brain through fast fibres that are non-nociceptive, and such novel *skin*information, novel *skin*put, can help a brain figure out a way to change, dissolve stalled movement that does not serve it well, that may have come from a spinal cord that has seniority in evolutionary terms, that can and will take over to protect its organism with default withdrawal reflex, my question is, why would we **not** want to take full advantage of such an easy way to treat pain and movement dysfunctions?

Contract-relax approach (some of the "neuro" in dermoneuromodulating)

In this approach, you recruit the patient to deploy a bit of motor output effort themselves, while you block any actual movement from happening.

Way back in physiotherapy school, long ago (late 1960's) I was taught contract-relax approach, along with a confused sort of reasoning that had to do with muscle testing and strengthening and trying to gain increases in range of motion by working muscle. The implication was that misbehaving muscles were causing pain. Later on, I learned that the exact same process could be applied to the spine, in order to get vertebrae that supposedly could not move by themselves for whatever reason, to move, by getting the patient to isolate and contract muscles that were attached to said vertebrae. The implication was that misbehaving joints were causing pain. However crude or incorrect that reasoning is from a modern pain/nerve perspective, the contract-relax approach itself does not hurt the person, and need not be applied overly-specifically. If you consider that nerves are 72 kilometers of passive noodle inside the body and skin organ, moving or pumping neural tunnels themselves makes sense, as new neurovascular physiology will be encouraged by such mechanical stimuli. As we probably all know by now, motion is lotion.

Positional relaxation approach (more of the "neuro" in dermoneuromodulating)

We have already mentioned that quadruped position may well remove much of the strain from a cranky peripheral nervous system.

Positioning may also be used to target specific portions of the neural tree, and the nerve itself may be moved specifically within its container. Michael Shacklock showed proof of concept for specificity of nerve movement in a video of a median nerve visualized by ultrasound. First the nerve is shown moving naturally, gliding back and forth along with the tendon moving the hand at the wrist. Then Michael moves his neck into lateral flexion away from his hand, and the nerve moves specifically, while the tendon (part of the nerve's "container") does not move. Thus, he showed that nerve movement and container movement can be differentiated. Recently he has gone on to show that contralateral movement can also affect an ipsilateral nerve. Thank you, Michael Shacklock.

Twizzling approach (more of the "neuro" in dermoneuromodulating)

Think of tie-rods in cars – they transmit forces along rods over considerable distance, from the steering wheel to the axles of a car, to turn the wheels. Think of a screwdriver. You twist the handle and a pivotal force goes down the axis of the bit to its end, and something on the end of the bit (the screw) is physically twisted.

In the human body, there is not likely to be any actual differentiated movement. However, there may be some sort of mild force that might move a nerve away or toward a vascular aspect nearby, in some deep part of the body, which is too deep to access any other way.

Everything in the body seems to be slightly spiralled – this probably adds strength and perhaps a degree of springiness to tissue without adding bulk. I have figured out ways (to try, at least) to "twizzle" nerves in their containers. "Twizzlers" are long, bendy ropes of candy, with longitudinal ridges that appear twisted around the rope. To twizzle, therefore, a verb in this treatment sense, is to rotate a nerve (or try to) around its longitudinal axis. Or, it could mean to try to rotate the container of the nerve around the longitudinal axis of the nerve.

Ordinary neurodynamics approaches are about positioning limbs, then bending distal appendages (hands or feet) into flexion and extension to glide long nerves through tunnels, or moving them by their central attachment at the spinal cord by moving the spine. I have added quadruped positioning, and an element of longitudinal rotation, with the idea that one might be able to rotate the container one way, and then longitudinally rotate the nerve the other way.

The "modulating" in dermoneuromodulating

This part is completely up to the person, brain, and nervous system you are involved with. Hopefully modulation will be in the direction both you and the patient would like it to go. But there is no way to know in advance what any individual nervous system will do, exactly. Create as advantageous a context for treatment as well as you can:

1. Provide a comfortable treatment setting.
2. Listen, listen, listen; ask questions gently, get all the details, let people express themselves, tell their story; do not interrupt.
3. When they are ready, provide pain education at the level they can take it in, and weave in relevant details they have provided to you.
4. Explain the treatment, make sure they understand they have locus of control, do not add any nocebo or nociception to them or their nerves.
5. Let treatment be slow enough to give their brain a chance to re-regulate and inhibit protective, defensive spinal cord processing.
6. Give them some movement homework; do not make promises (because you do not know exactly what their nervous system will do), but leave them with hope.

It is OK to tell them they should continue to improve for about 3 days following a treatment, because receptors will turn over in the ends of neurons to ones that are less sensitive; explain that continued improvement will be contingent on them doing their homework (any homework given should be easy and comfortable for them). Tell them, motion is lotion. Put them back in charge of care and feeding of any cranky nerves that you have discovered and treated together. Tell them that movement homework is like taking "move-better pills," to help their nerves get healthy again.

Homework may well include some change in asymmetric default resting positions, or asymmetric habitual behaviour, that you may have uncovered, as well – such as:

1. Always crossing one leg and never the other
2. Always sleeping on one side, never the other.

3. Always leaning on one elbow, never the other

4. Always standing on one leg with one hip jutted, never the other

5. Always carrying a heavy bag over one shoulder, never the other

6. Always carrying the baby on one hip, never the other

7. Always tucking one's feet to the side under the chair, always the same side

8. Etcetera.

We are doomed, most of us, to being asymmetric and doing things lopsidedly, because of having a dominant hand and eye. In my opinion, it does not matter *what* people *actively* do with their bodies, or how, as long as they move more: from the chest down, however, people might benefit a great deal by teaching themselves to organize their body and their peripheral neural tree more equitably, relative to gravity and load, by practicing all their ordinary default *resting* behaviours on the *other* side of themselves, about 50% of the time.

Now, onto treatment suggestions themselves.

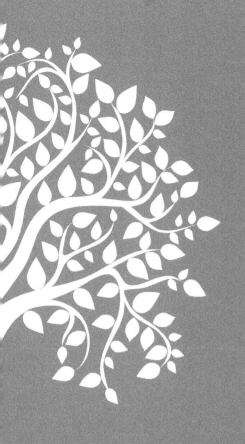
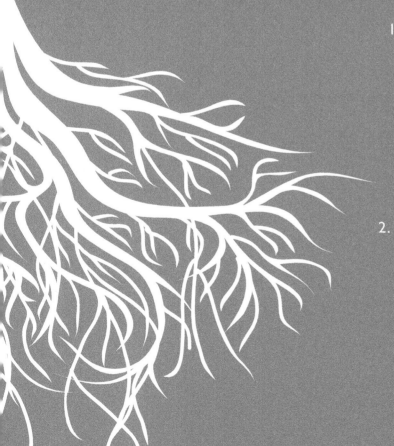

B. Treatment Section

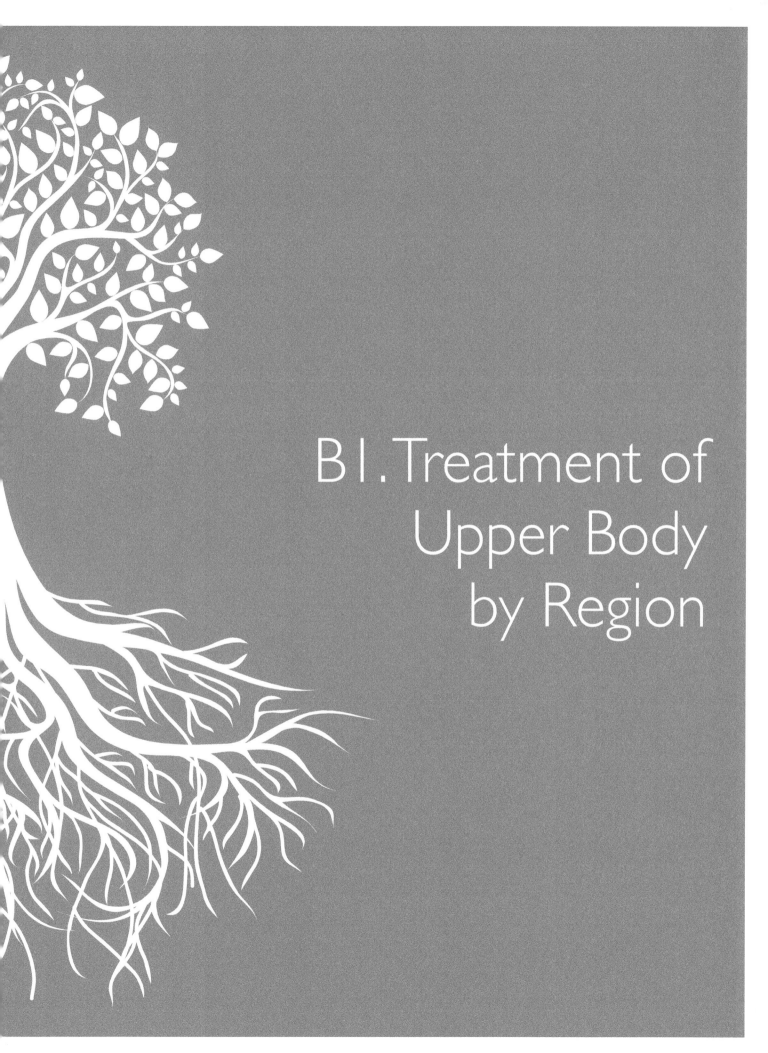

B1. Treatment of Upper Body by Region

HEAD AND NECK

Please note: Treatment suggestions for nerves of the face are beyond the scope of this book, which addresses spinal nerves.

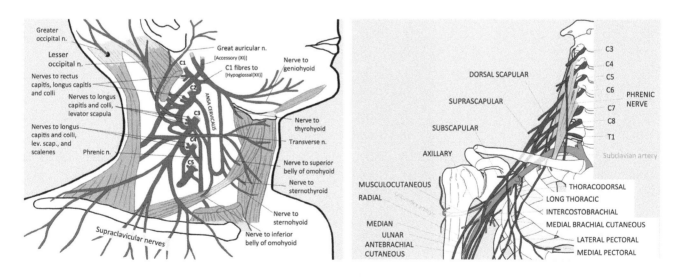

Cervical and brachial plexuses, and main nerves of the upper body.

HIGH NECK AND BACK OF HEAD

The dorsal ramus of C1 becomes Suboccipital nerve, motor to muscles that balance the head upon the neck. No part of it becomes cutaneous. It is best to address the occipital nerves, which are closer to the surface, first.

OCCIPITAL NERVES (C2):

C2 has massively branched dorsal rami, the **_greater occipital nerves_**, which become cutaneous, emerging in the neck and disseminating upward to supply all the skin over the back of the head.

The presentation will usually be associated with recent whiplash injury. The patient will usually have been medically cleared, but may be experiencing headache, sore stiff neck that feels worse when moving the neck, especially on forward flexion. The examiner will usually find fairly superficial, tender, sometimes palpably firm nodules at bottom edge of occiput, where occipital nerves surface into the skin organ. These nerves, like all nerves, vary from one individual to another; so will the sore spots. There will usually be at least one on each side, sometimes as many as three on each side.

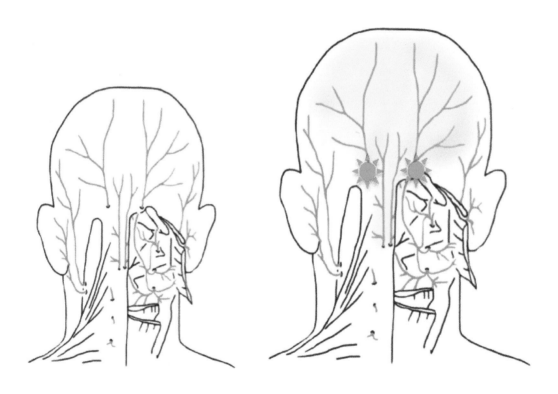

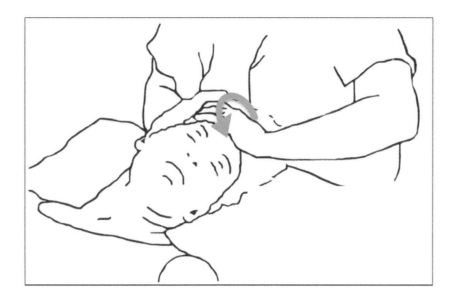

INDICATION: HEADACHE, TENDERNESS, LOSS OF RANGE OF MOTION

TREATMENT: POSITIONAL RELAXATION PLUS SKIN STRETCH APPROACH

1. Patient is supine. Legs are comfortably supported over a bolster. Arms are secured at sides of body so patient can let go easier. A pillow may be used, if necessary, but treating without one is easier.

2. Find first tender point, usually along occipital ridge short distance from midline, to right or left.

3. Position upper neck in slight extension, slight side bend *toward,* and slight rotation *away,* from side with tender point, to shorten and widen neural container.

4. Maintaining thumb contact, swivel non-monitoring hand upward to place it on skin over forehead.

5. Wait for your skin to stick to theirs, and then gently twist the skin slowly and carefully in the same direction their nose is pointing, until tender spot beneath monitoring hand softens and tenderness disappears.

6. Sometimes tenderness will not go completely. If you can get it to be 80% better it will usually go the rest of the way by itself. The patient will often palpably relax and their breathing deepen as soon as their tenderness feels relieved.

7. Hold that position for at least 2 minutes. Relinquish your hand position and force, slowly. Return head gently to neutral position.

8. Treat other spots if present in the same way.

9. Take out the bolster; support the patient to rise up to a sitting position so they can test their neck for improved comfort and range of movement. It is not uncommon for them to make comments related to improved interoception such as, "more space," "less compressed," "neck feels longer," "head feels lighter, like a helium balloon."

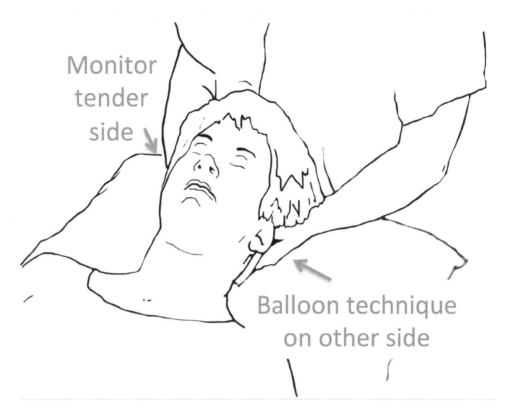

Monitor
tender
side

Balloon technique
on other side

TREATMENT VARIATION: SKIN STRETCH BALLOON APPROACH

1. Find tender spot.
2. Use other hand to treat, pulling skin into a "bunch" over the *other* occipital ridge. Go *slowly*.
3. Tender spot will usually soften and not be tender anymore.
4. Hold for at least 2 minutes.
5. Let go slowly

These two approaches will usually take care of any pain or tenderness or movement dysfunction that may be arising due to neural entrapment of cutaneous dorsal nerves, from C2. Now that we have the more superficial occipital nerves dealt with, we can go to the deeper and more complex suboccipital nerve from C1.

SUBOCCIPITAL NERVE (C1):

This nerve innervates all the muscles that attach head to neck. No part of it is cutaneous, so it cannot be moved directly. It may be *affected*, however, by moving

    a.   the parts that are connected by the muscles it innervates

    b.   which are, in turn, the nerve's containment system.

More about this, in a minute, but first, let us look at the anatomy a bit closer.

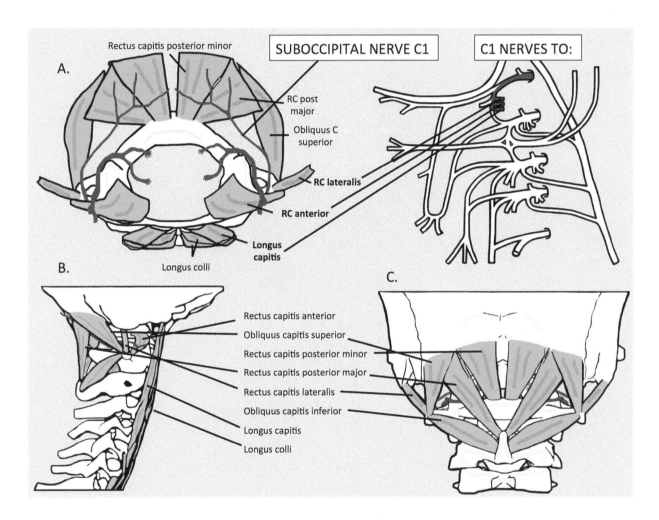

All the muscles supplied by suboccipital nerve: (A) view from above, looking down through the atlas; (B) lateral view; (C) posterior view

Great caution is recommended when moving the parts that constitute the high neck, as very important vasculature feeding the brain is situated there. Careful, interactive low velocity movement, such as we will discuss in a moment, is much safer than high velocity manipulation, because the brain will be able to monitor better via proprioceptive input and have more time to adapt its physiology to the applied forces.

Do not use direct pressure as a treatment tactic for any tenderness found in the region.

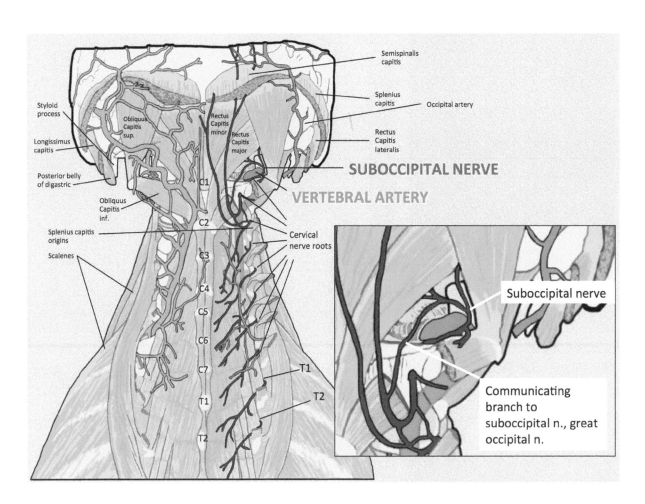

Neuroanatomy of the high neck. Note proximity of vertebral artery to suboccipital nerve, and note communicating branch between suboccipital nerve and occipital nerve.

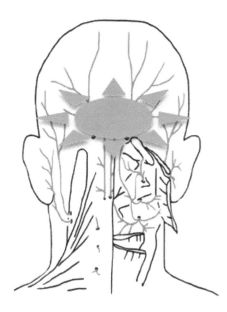

A person presents with a dull headache at the back of the head. They cannot flex their neck fully to tuck their chin to their chest. They may have had a recent fall in which their chin hit the ground, or hit something on the way down. They have been cleared medically for fracture of their odontoid process, or rheumatoid arthritis, or meningitis, a few of the major red flags that would make you not want to proceed.

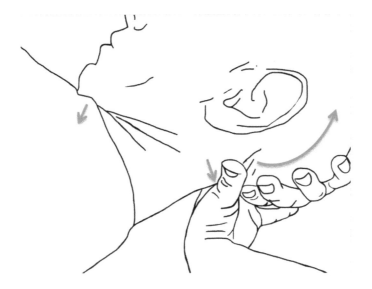

INDICATION: DULL HEADACHE BACK OF HEAD, INCREASED PAIN ON CHIN TUCK

TREATMENT: POSITIONAL RELAXATION COMBINED
WITH CONTRACT-RELAX APPROACH

1. Patient is supine, no pillow.

2. Reassure patient that you are *not* going to make any sudden moves, that you will go slow and explain what you are doing every step of the way, that they will be asked to contract a few muscles but that you will make it easy by supporting most of the weight of their head. Instruct them to tell you if they have any discomfort at any time. Meanwhile, watch their eyes carefully for any signs of discomfort and stay in verbal contact.

3. Slide your non-dominant hand carefully in behind top of neck to support the neck at the junction between head and neck, while you cradle head with other hand/arm. The support hand must be rigidly vertical; medial border of your hand on the bed, lateral border supporting the neck; use the strongest, thickest part of your hand, metacarpal phalangeal joints and webspace.

4. Bring the patient's head up into slight flexion. Ask patient to contract their chin toward their neck *while leaving their neck in contact with* your hand; continue to support of most of the weight of their head with your other hand.

5. After about 5 seconds, ask patient to relax. Take up any slack in range that now presents itself and maintain it.

6. Repeat twice more. After each repetition, take up slack in range.

7. Lower head gently down to treatment bed. Let the patient rest for a few moments.

8. Ask the patient to rise; have one hand behind their head to support it, and give them your other arm to help them pull up.

9. Check range of chin tuck in sitting. Usually it will have increased.

INDICATION: CHIN TUCK HAS IMPROVED BUT HIGH NECK
ROTATION IS STILL SLIGHTLY RESTRICTED OR PAINFUL

TREATMENT VARIATION: POSITIONAL RELAXATION COMBINED WITH
CONTRACT-RELAX APPROACH, INTO SLIGHT SIDE BEND AND ROTATION

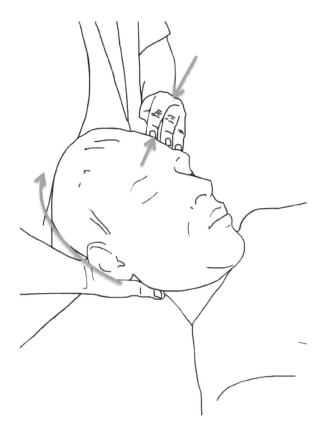

*One may view the zone between head and neck as somewhat analogous to a ball and
socket joint. Sometimes the sides need to be more specifically addressed.*

1. All the same handling tips as before apply to this variation.

2. Support neck on top on web space of one hand, at junction between head and neck.

3. Position head into slight flexion, slight side bend to left, slight rotation to right.

4. Support back of head in one hand. Place finger pads against forehead as shown.

5. Ask patient to press head slightly against the fingers, upward with the corner of their forehead, diagonally, for about 5 seconds.

6. Upon relaxation, some increased slack usually occurs. Take it up carefully.

7. Repeat twice more.

8. Treat other side also.

INDICATION: DISCOMFORT AND/OR SLIGHT RESTRICTION ON ROTATION

TREATMENT VARIATION: POSITIONAL RELAXATION COMBINED WITH
DIRECT PRESSURE FROM OPPOSITE SIDE, TO UNLOAD FROM WITHIN

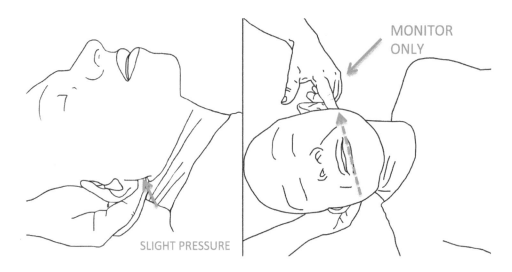

Once in awhile the first two technique suggestions simply do not take care of all of it. The pain will be felt more laterally, closer to the ear. If you press in with your little finger, directly below the ear, between the mastoid process and the angle of the jaw, there may be a sharply tender spot on one side compared to the other, or sometimes both sides. Choose the more tender side to treat first.

1. Locate tender point in neck just below the ear.
2. Monitor with one finger.
3. Move head into slight extension, side bend and rotation away, as shown.
4. Find the opposite C1 transverse process and carefully, slowly press into it, as though you were sliding it or shearing it diagonally sideways a little bit, up toward the tender point side.
5. Tenderness in the tender side will disappear.
6. Maintain this minimum necessary pressure (i.e., don't add any *more* pressure), for about 90 seconds. Be sure patient is comfortable throughout.
7. You should be able to feel a growing sense of relief and relaxation within the neck itself, as you wait. If you do not feel this, ask your patient if you are creating any discomfort for them. If you are, shift your angle slightly.
8. Slowly let go, bring your patient's neck and head into neutral, allow them to rest for a few moments, then help them to sit up, let them check their movement.

DermoNeuroModulating | Diane Jacobs

POSTERIOR NECK

DORSAL RAMI: Most of us have probably seen examples of animal mothers transporting their young, carrying them by the scruff of the neck. The animal infants relax completely, and the mothers appear to be very gentle with their use of jaws and teeth for this purpose.

The back of the neck is very easy to treat, by simply attending to the dorsal cutaneous rami there. In fact, all the dorsal cutaneous rami all the way down the back are easy to treat, but for now, we will only address the ones that serve the back of the neck.

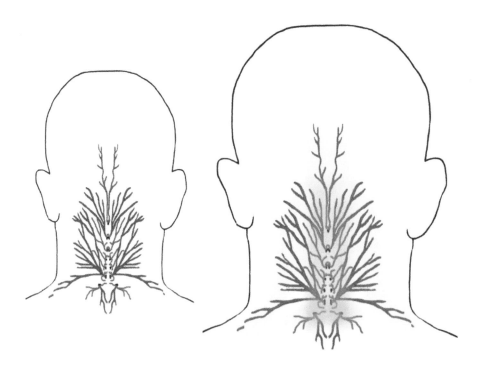

The dorsal rami help to innervate all the neck muscles that lie behind the transverse processes. Their cutaneous branches supply the skin with sensory and autonomic innervation.

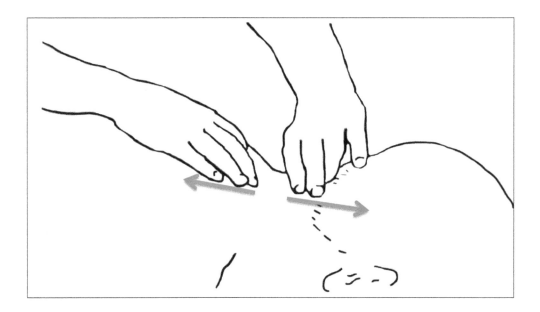

TREATMENT: SKIN STRETCHING APPROACH

1. Patient is prone. A face hole in the bed, padded for complete comfort, is essential. A head-piece, hinged so that it may be dropped down as necessary to position neck in a bit of flexion, is ideal.

2. Place fingers along spinous processes landmarks, wait for your finger pads to "stick" to patient's skin

3. The diagram shows the skin being stretched longitudinally (parallel to spine, and near to spinous processes) in directions shown – caudal and cephalad

4. The skin can be stretched in any direction however; diagonally, clockwise, counterclockwise be creative. Go with whatever seems a direction of ease.

5. Hold for 2 minutes. Take up any slack as it presents itself.

6. Let go slowly.

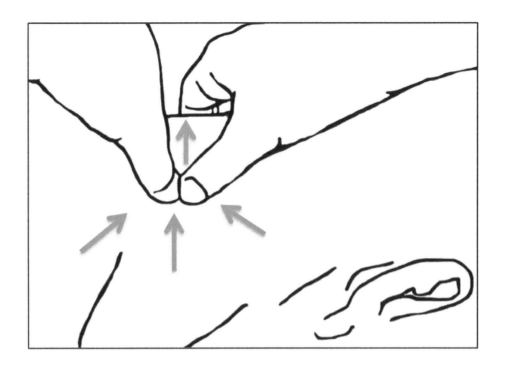

TREATMENT VARIATION: SKIN STRETCH COMBINED WITH
BALLOON APPROACH "KITTEN TECHNIQUE"

1. Place both hands gently upon the back of neck in wide grasp. Wait for hands to stick to skin.

2. Slowly, gently, pull skin layer up toward ceiling. All tissues connected to skin organ, suspended from within, will be dragged upward as well.

3. Hold for at least 2 minutes, longer as required. You should be able to feel a sense of relaxation occur within the neck, and spread to include the whole person. As always, especially regarding anything to do with neck, do not press, and monitor patient closely.

4. Gently lower the skin down, and remove hands from neck.

5. Ask patient to stand up and reassess neck movement and comfort level.

SUPERFICIAL CERVICAL PLEXUS: The first thing one notices about the side of the neck, is the main muscle in that neighbourhood, sternocleidomastoid. I urge you to forget about SCM as a treatment target; digging into it with your fingers is *not* recommended. Instead consider it as a useful landmark. What IS important is that a large plexus of cutaneous neural array, the superficial cervical plexus, lying directly on top of it. Just moving the skin over SCM easily moves this plexus.

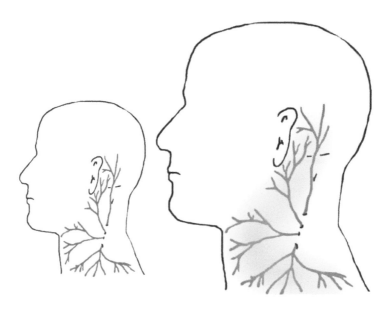

A bit of anatomical orientation: the area between SCM and the clavicle forms a triangle; the sternal notch is the medial corner. This zone is called, predictably, the "anterior triangle." Generally, I have found that best results are gained when skin within the triangle is moved toward the sternal notch.

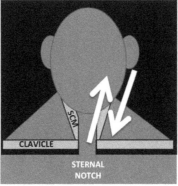

Move skin within anterior triangle toward notch

ANTERIOR TRIANGLE OF NECK

So, to treat superficial cervical plexus, use SCM as a landmark, and slide the skin along its borders.

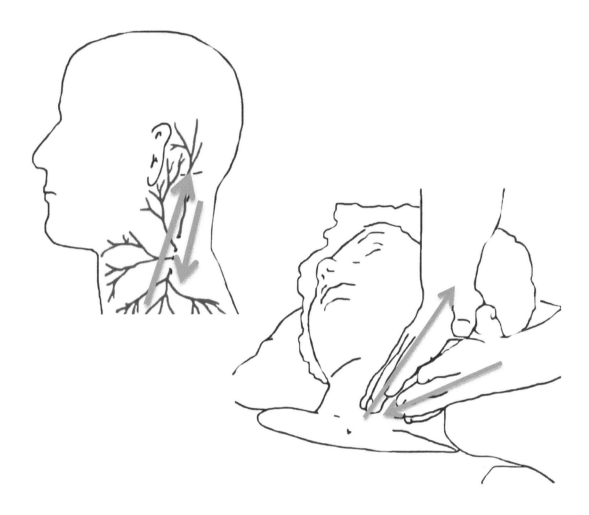

INDICATION: NECK PAIN, STIFFNESS, RESTRICTED NECK ROTATION

TREATMENT: SKIN STRETCH APPROACH

1. Patient is supine.
2. Turn head slightly to one side, so there is room for your hands.
3. Place medial borders of your hands on skin above and below SCM.
4. Wait for your hands to "attach" to patient's skin
5. Slowly and carefully, slide the skin in the directions shown.
6. Hold for about 2 minutes. You should be able to feel softening begin to occur fairly rapidly. When it feels like it stops...
7. Let go slowly.
8. Help your patient sit up, and reassess rotation. Often there will be a good deal more of it available.
9. Treat the other side if necessary.

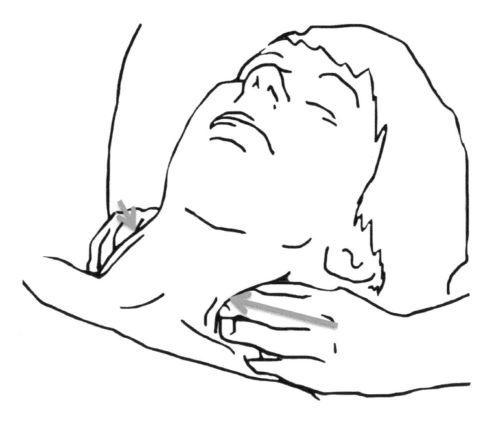

TREATMENT VARIATION: SKIN STRETCH APPROACH

1. Patient is supine
2. Place ends of finger gently in under SCM landmark, on top of transverse processes. (Do not press down.)
3. Wait for your skin to "attach" to patient's skin
4. Slowly and carefully, slide the skin in the directions shown. Be slow and very gentle. Again, do not press down – instead, "lift" the tissues up slightly with the backs of your fingers. Check in with how this feels to your patient; it should feel weirdly interesting and relieving to the patient. (If your patient says they feel as though they have black spots in front of their eyes, you are pressing instead of lifting - get off their carotid arteries right away!)
5. Hold for about 2 minutes. Let go slowly. Remove fingers gently.

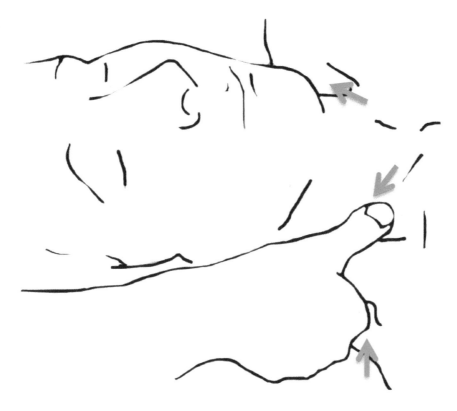

TREATMENT VARIATION: BALLOON APPROACH - BILATERAL
OR UNILATERAL GRASP WITH SKIN STRETCH

1. Patient supine

2. Loosely grasp skin over SCM on both sides

3. Wait for your skin to "attach" to patient's skin

4. Slowly and carefully, pull the skin into your grasp. Don't pinch. Be slow and very gentle. This is like the "kitten technique" we saw previously for the posterior neck. Be much lighter in grasping skin here on the sides of the neck.

5. Hold for about 2 minutes. Slight torque may be added if it feels as though it adds increased relaxation.

6. Let go slowly.

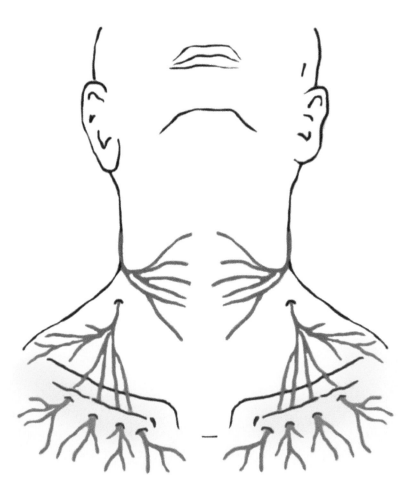

SUPRACLAVICULAR NERVES: Part of the superficial cervical plexus array is a wide dissemination of supraclavicular nerves; like a very large collar, these nerves supply skin over, down, and across the chest, over the shoulders, and over the tops of the shoulders down a little way over the posterior shoulder girdle.

The nerves themselves must cross within the skin over the clavicles through narrow tunnels, where they can get into some problems. When a patient comes in with neck pain, restricted rotation, and rounded looking shoulders, it might be prudent to investigate these nerves.

Here is a picture of the anterior triangle again.

Move skin within anterior
triangle toward notch

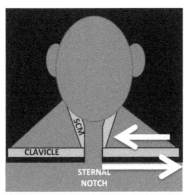

ANTERIOR TRIANGLE OF NECK

Moving skin gently and slowly in directions shown by arrows seems to work best.

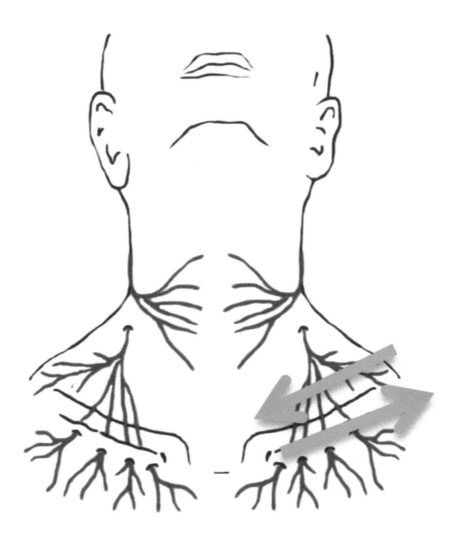

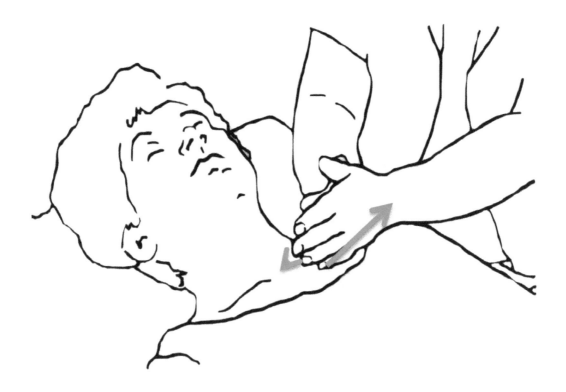

INDICATION: NECK PAIN, HEADACHE, ROUND-SHOULDERED
APPEARANCE, SHOULDERS PULLED UP

TREATMENT: SKIN STRETCH APPROACH

1. Patient is supine.
2. Place medial borders of hands on skin above and below clavicle landmark.
3. Wait for your skin to "attach" to patient's skin
4. Slowly and carefully, slide the skin in the directions shown.
5. Hold for about 2 minutes
6. Let go slowly
7. If this was the right treatment, upon reexamination, you will notice the shoulders will appear more squared, easily sit further back, and the patient can rotate their neck easier.

ANTERIOR SHOULDER

We are now moving laterally, to the fronts of the shoulders. People often feel pain at the fronts of shoulders. I think that often pain felt here has nothing at all to do with any deep structure in the region, just nerves, often branches of these same nerves we have just discussed.

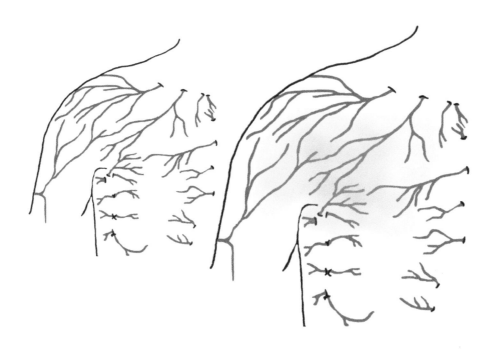

Cutaneous nerves commonly anastomose. In front of the shoulder, supraclavicular cutaneous nerves, from C3, branching downward and outward, may be anastomosed with (a) branches of lateral cutaneous nerve of the arm, from C5, branching upward and medially and/or (b) branches of intercostobrachial nerve from T2, coming upward from axilla. You just never know. But these are possibilities, and where nerves join up, neural tunnel problems may become more complicated when tugged.

We are going to take a detour at this point: we will return to anterior shoulder after examining cutaneous nerves in the upper back, around the sides of the trunk, and inferior shoulder.

NECK AND UPPER BACK

DORSAL RAMI: We need to take a brief moment to talk about ***dorsal rami***. Dorsal rami nerves are generally shorter and more regular, more segmental, whereas ventral rami do all sorts of complex crisscrossing by forming plexuses, are way longer, and are responsible for innervating way more of the body.

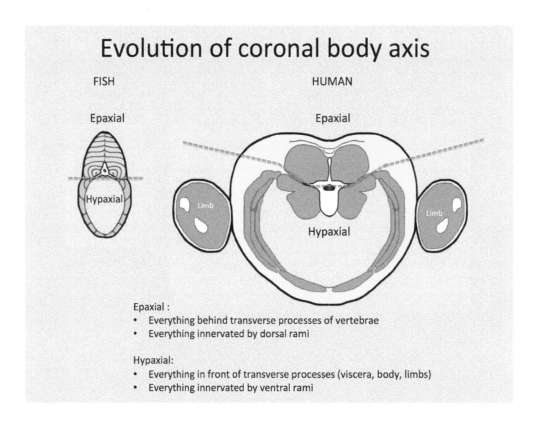

View is from the top down, a coronal view. All the musculature behind the transverse process is termed "epaxial"; all the musculature in front of the transverse processes is termed "hypaxial." As you can see, ventral innervation expanded a lot over evolutionary time.

Dermoneuromodulation | Diane Jacobs

When our fish ancestors became vertebrates, they evolved the spinal cord with a flexible bony column to protect it. They were supported by and swam around in water. They used their whole body, horizontally, with side-to-side sinusoidal movement, and likely used their fins just for steering and maybe sensing.

Their spinal nerves divided immediately upon exiting the spinal canal: dorsal rami innervated the musculature on their backs, and ventral rami innervated musculature on their fronts. Both sets of musculature were about equal in size. This division of labour worked out very well.

Fish ancestors eventually came out onto land, and evolved into animals that grew legs. Large foreleg muscles grew over top of the muscles that were still innervated by dorsal rami. Although we are no longer quadrupeds, we still have latissimus dorsi, a foreleg muscle that is now an arm muscle. It is innervated mainly by ventral rami, the ***thoracodorsal nerve*** from the brachial plexus, but covers almost the entire back, attached firmly to the spine from T6 all the way down to the end of the sacrum! The cutaneous branches of dorsal rami have to be mobile inside tunnels *through* all that, all the way down. (They also help innervate it, send small branches into it, close to the spine.)

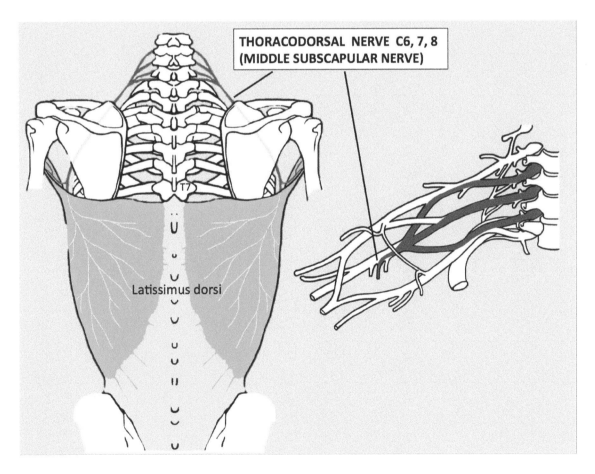

Lat dorsi muscle and thoracodorsal nerve

We still have muscles innervated only by dorsal rami; they lie deeply buried, directly against the spine. A simple rule is, if it is segmental muscle, and behind the transverse processes, it will be innervated by dorsal rami. (Another rule seems to be, the smaller the muscle, the longer its name! but I digress.)

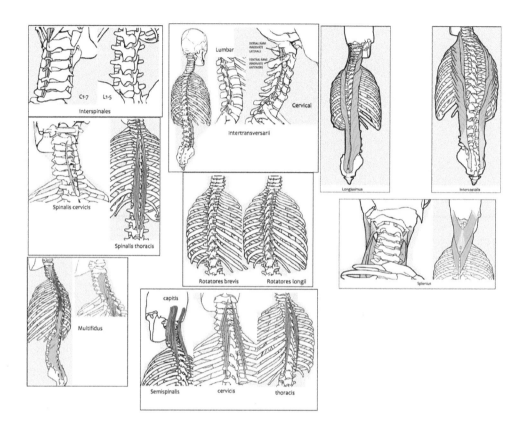

All the musculature innervated by motor branches of dorsal rami. All other musculature in our musculoskeletal system is innervated by ventral rami, including all limb muscle.

Cutaneous branches of dorsal rami are much longer and more extensively disseminated than are motor branches. Furthermore, they are extensively overlapped and anastomosed as well.

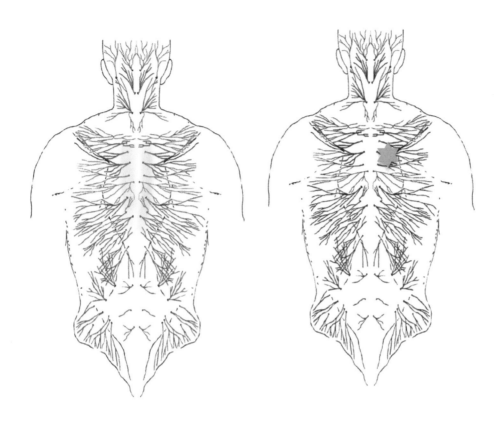

Cutaneous dorsal rami are everywhere across the back of the shoulders and shoulder girdle. Interscapular pain is a common problem.

Most of us have a dominant hand and arm; non-symmetrical use of the shoulder girdle is practically a given. A patient who comes to see you with interscapular pain is likely to have fallen into fairly extreme asymmetrical habits or use, often over a lifetime. Maybe they have carried their bag on one side exclusively all their lives, or currently carry a young child, usually just on one hip, not the other. Maybe they have leaned over on the same elbow for years, or decades. Maybe they only ever sleep on one side. It is good to assess their posture but do not make any sort of big deal out of it or blame their structure – posture is just a snapshot in time. Delicately extract as much information from people as you can about how they inhabit their physicality, and help them to understand why habits and default resting positions may take a toll or contribute to a pain experience. They may be completely unaware of how they use/misuse their body and might never have put such clues together on their own. It is important to stress that it is not "damage" or even their fault and that learning new habits will not be impossible or even hard, and will not even take very long.

INDICATION: NAGGING LOWER NECK, OR THORACIC PAIN: "NOTALGIA PARESTHETICA"

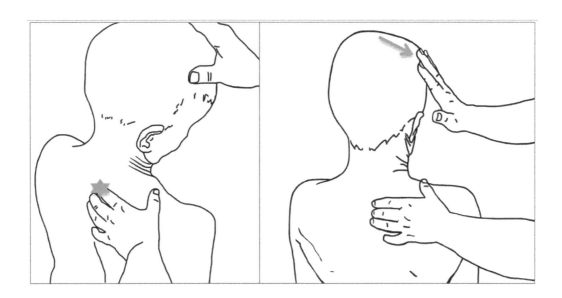

TREATMENT: CONTRACT-RELAX APPROACH

1. Patient is seated. With one hand, contact the skin over the area with tenderness. With other hand, guide the patient's head and neck slowly and carefully into a combination of flexion (or extension), side bend, and rotation (toward, usually, but it might be away), any combination that provides the best unloading of the area and relief for the patient. The perfect combination will be any position in which you feel the area "move" slightly beneath your sensitive fingers. Ask the patient to stay right there.

2. Place your hand against patient's head. Ask patient to press slightly against your hand, in that direction, without moving your hand. After 5-10 seconds, ask them to relax ask them to relax. This is an isotonic contraction initiated by them, even though they will not physically move anywhere, which means it is isometric as well. It works better, probably for "locus of control" reasons, to ask the patient to contract against your resistance, rather than asking them to hold while you push against them. In any case, the amount of pressure needed is very minimal.

3. You will notice this creates a bit of space, or softening, in the area of concern.

4. Find the next position, and repeat, for total of three times.

It is plausible that active contraction of musculature in the region pulls against the neural tunnels, opening up more space for the dorsal ramus at all levels, not just superficially, and also provides a novel stimulus to the nervous system. Occasionally a great deal of heat is thrown off the affected area in the process of getting it to move, perhaps the first time the patient has moved that particular place in a long time.

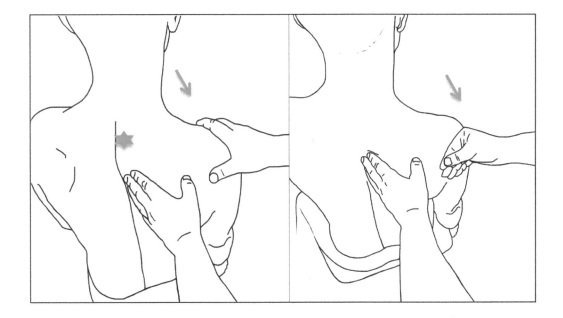

The same approach may be used further down the back, by having the patient press their shoulder against your hand instead of their head.

The beauty of this approach is that it takes very little effort from the patient, and can be used anywhere in three-dimensional space, at any angle of flexion *or* extension, combined with side bend and rotation. With a bit of practice anyone can become adept at such three-dimensional positioning of a willing patient. Patients like it because it does not hurt them, and they feel more in control.

If you want the patient to be able to move further into flexion, provide them a platform against which they can press (no image available):

1. Ask them to bend their elbows, cross their arms to hold opposite elbows, lift their elbows up in front.

2. Reach your own arm around their trunk, beneath their elbows, and place your hand against their back, or side of their trunk, opposite you

3. They now have a platform against which they can actively contract into flexion, rotation and side bend, while you provide them resistance.

For more specifically cutaneous neural entrapments, you need a different strategy. The patient needs to be as relaxed as possible, not contracting anything.

INDICATION: PERSISTING PAIN FELT ANYWHERE
BESIDE SPINE, BETWEEN C7 and T12.

TREATMENT: SKIN STRETCH APPROACH

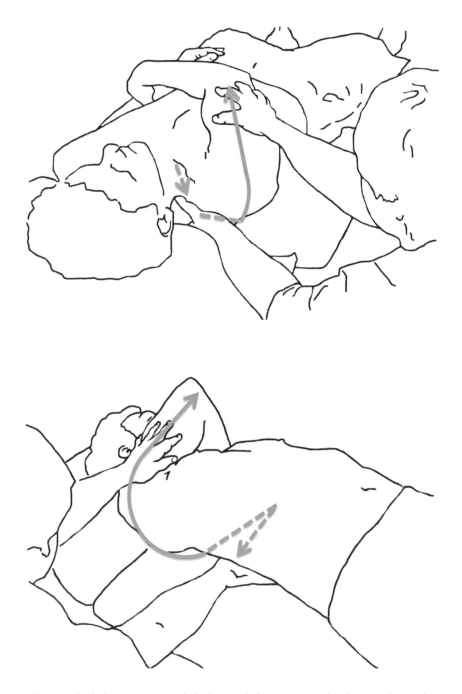

The degree of arc available for treatment. Pick the best angle for treatment of each particular tender spot found.

1. Patient is supine, legs up and comfortably supported by a bolster.

2. Slide you hand under patient, find their spine, and then come off it slightly onto the muscular prominence. Your patient is supported in, and by, gravity, so tension is not required by their nervous system. Therefore any palpable tension may be considered a 'sign'. Locate a sore spot in the near vicinity – monitor it with one hand.

3. With your other hand elevate patient's arm on same side. Move the arm in an arc across their body, until you feel something move or soften slightly at your monitoring hand under the patient. That will be the perfect angle to begin treating. Place the arm over the patient at that angle.

4. Move your outside hand to the skin on the back of the patient's arm, and draw it carefully but inexorably toward the patient's elbow, taking care to not press patient's entire arm into more adduction. You will feel the spinal area move under your monitoring hand. The muscle will immediately soften.

5. Hold for about two minutes. With monitoring hand, pull skin away from spine laterally if that improves the softening.

6. Let go slowly.

7. Ask patient to stand, move about, perform range of movement testing, to confirm/consolidate improvement.

LATERAL TRUNK AND INFERIOR SHOULDER

LATERAL CUTANEOUS NERVES OF THE TRUNK: We now turn our attention to *lateral cutaneous nerves of the trunk*. These are very, very long. They branch at a very sharp angle, into an anterior branch that runs forward to almost the front of the body, which may be anastomosed into anterior cutaneous nerves, and a posterior branch that reaches back, which may be anastomosed into dorsal cutaneous nerves. If you have ever experienced a "stitch" in your side after running, or felt that you "split your sides" by laughing really hard, it will likely be one of these nerves complaining, usually right at the "grommet hole" along the side of the body where it surfaces, before splitting into its anterior and posterior branches. Most of the time pain will not be felt directly at the sides; the grommet holes of these nerves are almost always tender, though, and the skin they innervate ticklish.

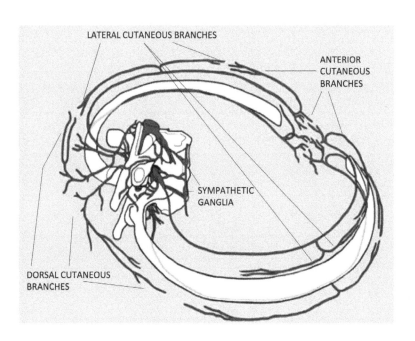

Dermoneuromodulation | Diane Jacobs

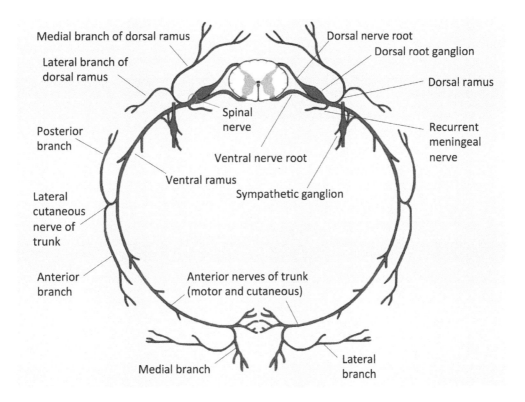

Medial branch of dorsal ramus

Lateral branch of dorsal ramus

Posterior branch

Lateral cutaneous nerve of trunk

Anterior branch

Spinal nerve

Ventral nerve root

Ventral ramus

Sympathetic ganglion

Dorsal nerve root

Dorsal root ganglion

Dorsal ramus

Recurrent meningeal nerve

Anterior nerves of trunk (motor and cutaneous)

Medial branch

Lateral branch

Note the combined length of lateral and anterior cutaneous nerves (ventral rami) compared to dorsal cutaneous rami.

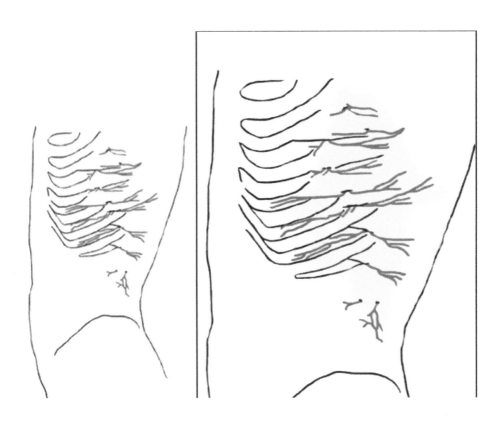

INDICATION: DULL BACK PAIN ANYWHERE ON ONE SIDE OF BACK BENEATH
OR INFERIOR TO SHOULDER BLADE, OVER RIB CAGE, OR PAINLESS
BUT RESTRICTED TRUNK SIDEBEND OR SHOULDER ELEVATION

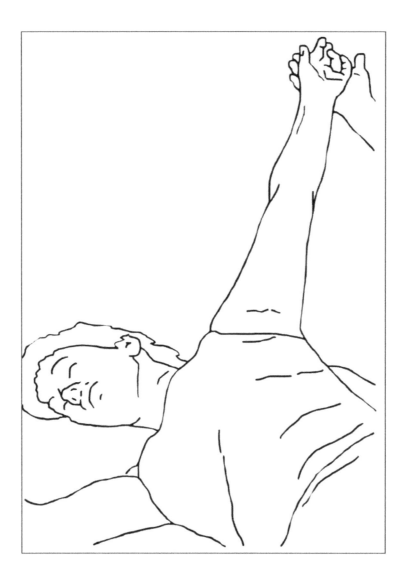

ASSESSMENT:

1. Patient is comfortable in sidelying.
2. Lift up the arm, slowly and carefully; take it up and back into abduction elevation until slight resistance is felt: This represents the limit of range.
3. **NB**: DO NOT EXCEED THIS FIRST SMALL BARRIER TO MOVEMENT

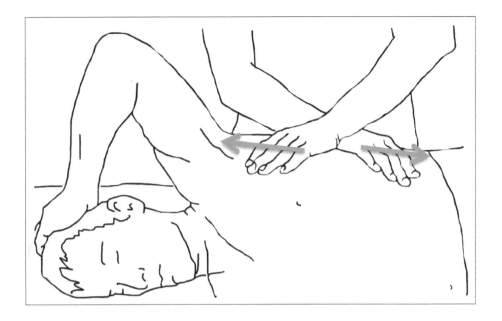

TREATMENT: SKIN STRETCH APPROACH

1. Ask patient to rest hand on top of forehead, and keep elbow up in the air

2. Place hands gently on side of trunk. Wait until hands stick to skin.

3. Gently lengthen the skin between two hands until slight resistance is encountered. Then wait for a few minutes.

4. Gently allow hands and skin under hands to come back to neutral. Remove hands slowly.

5. Carefully bring the patient's arm down to their side and let it rest for a moment.

6. Reassess*. Arm will usually be able to elevate much further, and more smoothly. The ribcage should be able to adapt more easily to the movement of the shoulder and individual ribs slide easier beneath the skin.

7. Ask patient to stand up and move to gauge any increase in comfort, perform trunk sidebend to see if it has increased, see if they can elevate arm more easily.

*TREATMENT TIP: When you reassess arm by lifting it, notice if it pulls either forward or backward. If it pulls forward you may need to treat nerves of anterior shoulder. If it pulls backward, you may need to treat nerves of posterior shoulder.

INTERCOSTOBRACHIAL NERVE: This is a good place to introduce you to a nerve that almost no one ever considers, the *intercostobrachial nerve*.

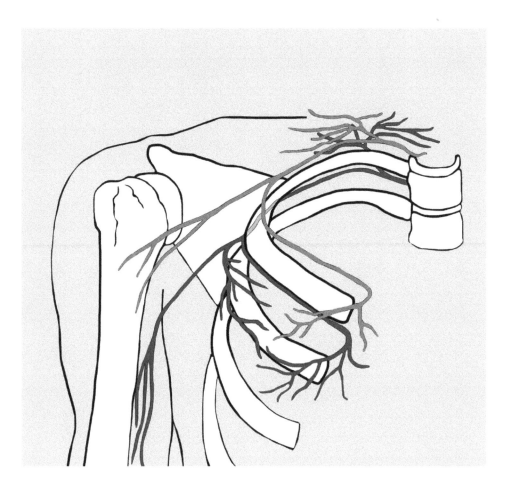

Intercostobrachial nerve from T2 in green. T1 spinal nerve shown in grey.

It is spinal nerve T2. It is an "orphan" nerve, because it is not truly typical as a spinal nerve, nor is it included in the brachial plexus with T1. It comes around the body the same way all the other spinal nerves do, but finds its way blocked by the presence of an arm. It emerges and divides into anterior and posterior branches at the axilla. It supplies the skin of the axilla. While the anterior branch continues around to the front of the body under the arm, the posterior branch goes down the inside of the arm toward the elbow. Heart attack can refer pain to this nerve, often, in the left arm. The posterior branch is often anastomosed into the medial cutaneous nerve of the arm, from T1.

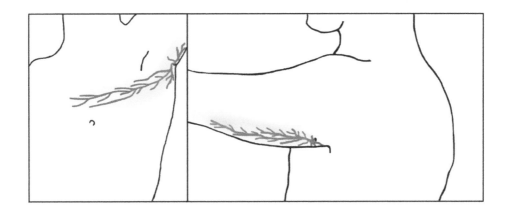

The anterior branch around chest wall, and posterior branch down arm.

One can treat this nerve easily with exactly the same assessment, and set up.

A bonus is that scapula makes a good handle; you can also move deeply buried motor nerves from the cervical and brachial plexus that supply any muscle connected to the scapula. This includes ***dorsal scapular nerve***, ***suprascapular nerve***, ***subscapular nerves***, ***thoracodorsal nerve***, ***long thoracic nerve***, and possibly the nerves to the two bellies of omohyoid (which attaches to the top medial corner of the scapula), and even (to a limited extent) accessory nerve to trapezius.

INDICATION: PERSISTING NON-MEDICAL CHEST PAIN,
PAIN DOWN BACK OR INSIDE OF ARM.

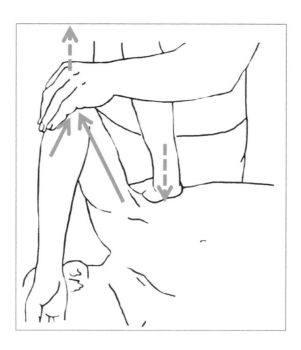

TREATMENT: SKIN STRETCH APPROACH COMBINED WITH
DIRECT PRESSURE ON LATERAL BORDER OF SCAPULA

1. Patient is in comfortable sidelying. You have performed the assessment previously described.
2. Place one hand gently over lateral border of scapula. Place other hand over entire elbow
3. Gently but inexorably press to move the scapula medially. Go slow. Wait for ease to present itself.
4. At the same time, gather the skin over the elbow up into the other hand, as if you were trying to pull it up toward the ceiling. A piece of dycem comes in very handy for this job as it is sticky and gives one better grip of skin, especially if your hands are small. This pulls the posterior branch of intercostobrachial nerve further out of its "grommet hole."
5. Hold for a few minutes.
6. Gently allow hands, and skin under hands, to come back to neutral. Remove hands slowly.
7. Reassess. Ask patient to stand up and move their arm around, perform range of motion through their trunk. Usually ribcage pain will feel greatly relieved.

AXILLARY NERVE: Another nerve in the vicinity, that can limit shoulder range and be very sore, is the *axillary nerve*. It is from the brachial plexus. It supplies deltoid muscle, and has a cutaneous branch wrapping around the top of the arm, called *lateral cutaneous nerve of the arm*. It has to exit through something called the "quadrangular space," bordered by teres major, teres minor, long head of triceps and the shaft of humerus. Not a lot of room - it can become scissored in there. The treatment set-up is a bit complex at first and will require some practice.

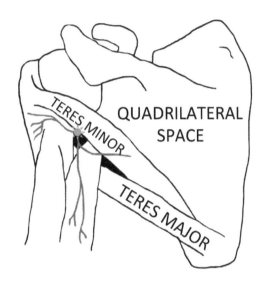

Quadrangular space

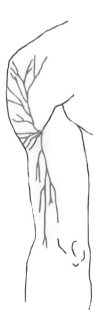

Posterior upper arm, lateral cutaneous nerve of arm.

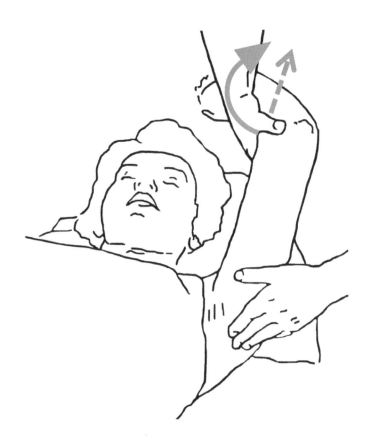

TREATMENT: POSITIONAL RELAXATION APPROACH, COMBINED
WITH SLIGHT TRACTION AND SKIN STRETCH

1. Bring arm gently up into about 90 degrees flexion at shoulder, 90 degrees of flexion at elbow, and about 45 degrees of internal rotation at shoulder, as shown. (When the arm is in correct position, the hand should be almost directly over the forehead.)

2. Hold patient's forearm with one hand, and locate sore spot at posterior axilla with the other. (Monitor only.) Upper arm remains vertical throughout.

3. With supporting hand, torque the skin of the forearm into *more* internal rotation, *plus,* lift the entire arm up slightly toward ceiling, unloading the sore spot at the posterior axilla.

4. Sore spot will soften and tenderness will disappear. After tenderness has disappeared, hold arm in this position for at least 2 minutes to ensure their brain has time to compute the new input successfully.

5. Slowly lower arm to side.

6. Ask patient to stand up and move arm around, perform range of motion. Pain on movement is usually gone.

POSTERIOR AND SUPERIOR SHOULDER

SUPRASCAPULAR NERVE: The suprascapular nerve is part of the brachial plexus, mostly C5 and 6. Part of the journey on its way to innervate the supraspinatus and infraspinatus muscles is to slide through and bend around a narrow fibro-osseous tunnel through the spine of the shoulder blade.

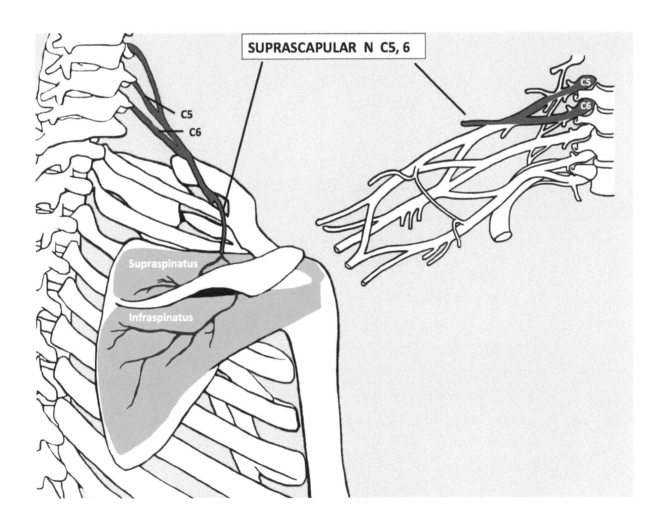

The sort of behaviour that might bother it over a lifetime includes carrying a heavy bag on the same shoulder all the time, repeated use of one arm to wield a heavy tool overhead, etc. There might be dull aching pain, sometimes a sharply tender spot, at the top of the spinous process of the scapula.

It is a motor nerve with no cutaneous branch to be able to affect directly with skin stretch, but it can be addressed indirectly by shortening and widening its neural tunnel as best you can, thereby slacking the nerve itself, and handling the arm carefully.

There is, of course, the posterior branch of the supraclavicular nerve lying over top of the area, which also will be affected by the treatment.

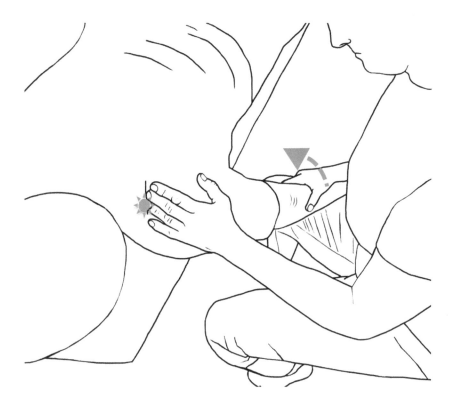

INDICATION: DULL PAIN AT TOP OR BACK OF SHOULDER,
POSSIBLY AN AREA OF TENDERNESS

TREATMENT: POSITIONAL RELAXATION APPROACH

1. Patient is prone with arm hanging freely.
2. Locate tender spot, if there is one. If not, palpate for something that feels too tight so you can position arm to help it soften.
3. Bring arm into about 45 degrees of extension, abduction and elevation from hanging, elbow straight. Rest it against knee.
4. Grasp forearm gently. Carefully torque it into slight external rotation. Tenderness will disappear immediately; softening will occur immediately. Hold for 2 minutes.
5. Slowly let go. Have patient stand up and reassess range of movement.

DermoNeuroModulating | Diane Jacobs

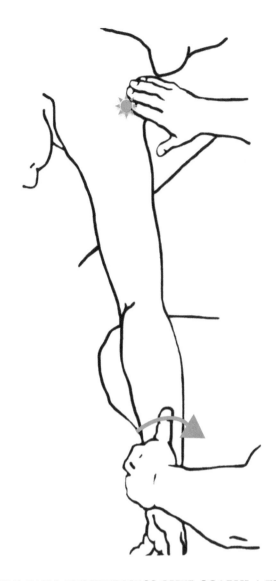

INDICATION: DULL PAIN, TENDERNESS OVER SCAPULA FURTHER CAUDAL

TREATMENT: POSITIONAL RELAXATION APPROACH

1. Patient is prone with arm hanging freely.
2. Take arm into about 45 degrees of flexion, abduction and elevation from hanging, elbow straight. Rest it on knee.
3. Locate tender spot over scapula. Do not press.
4. With other hand gently grasp skin over medial forearm, allow to stick, and torque forearm slowly into external rotation.
5. Sore spot will soften and tenderness will disappear. Hold arm in this position for at least 2 minutes.
6. Slowly let go and let arm hang freely. Reassess sore spot. It should be gone.
7. Ask patient to stand up and move their own arm around, perform range of motion.

POSTERIOR BRANCH OF SUPRACLAVICULAR NERVE

Tops of shoulders are famous for harbouring palpable "knots." These are uncomfortable, usually, but not especially painful. Everyone loves a good shoulder squeeze from friends they trust. Once in awhile though, these "knots" become painful, and do not respond to mere squeezing, or even to pressure by those trained in massage. At that point a more sophisticated approach may be necessary. Instead of thinking about loading, about squeezing muscle, we may need to shift toward thinking about unloading nerve structure. Nerves involved may be **accessory**, or **posterior branch of supraclavicular**, or a **dorsal ramus**, or any combination thereof.

INDICATION: A PAINFUL "KNOT" AT TOP OF SHOULDER

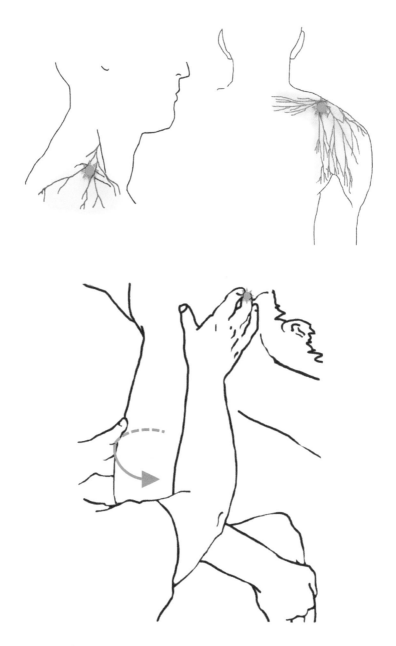

TREATMENT: POSITIONAL RELAXATION PLUS SKIN STRETCH APPROACH

1. Patient is prone. Arm is hanging freely.

2. Sit at side of table. Bend elbow to 90 degrees flexion, and rest it on knee. This gives you good control of shoulder. Pushing up slightly with your knee will lift the arm up vertically, taking all strain away from its suspension system, and will allow you to shorten and widen neural tunnels at the shoulder, if necessary. A variation is to simply continue to allow arm to hang freely. Choose whichever way works best for your patient.

3. Locate spot.

4. Gently grasp skin on back of arm. After hand has stuck to skin, slowly and gently drag the skin around into internal rotation.

5. Sore spot will soften and tenderness will go away. Hold for 2 minutes.

6. Let go slowly.

7. Ask patient to get up and move, perform range of motion.

DORSAL SCAPULAR NERVE

Dorsal scapular nerve is from the brachial plexus, mostly C5, with contributions from C3 and 4. It innervates levator scapulae and rhomboids.

If you have a patient with interscapular pain and/or tension that has not responded to treatment for dorsal rami, consider treatment for dorsal scapular nerve to see if it will help.

There may or may not be a tender spot.

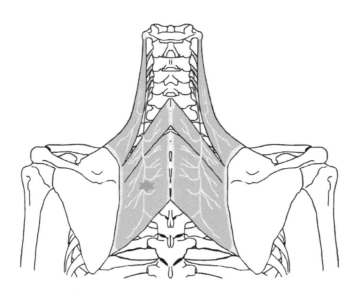

INDICATION: INTERSCAPULAR BACK PAIN

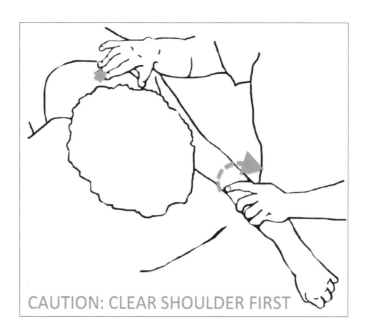

TREATMENT: POSITIONAL RELAXATION APPROACH

1. Patient is prone. Locate sore spot – monitor it with one hand
2. Place arm on same side into full elevation. Lift arm just up off the bed.
3. Take the skin layer of forearm into slight internal, or external, rotation – whichever works best for that individual.
4. Wait for softening, and then hold for a few minutes.
5. Let go slowly.
6. Ask patient to stand, move about, perform range of movement testing, to confirm/consolidate improvement

---

ACROMIOCLAVICULAR RETE

This is a good place to discuss retes in general, and the acromioclavicular rete in particular. The word "rete" comes from the Latin word for "net." Retes are tangled nets of interconnected vascular and neural structure, usually small diameter and dense, existing over bony prominences everywhere in the body. They do not have any specific direction. They permit the care and feeding of tissue even when it is stretched over an elbow, a trochanter, knee, a heel or an acromion process. Always ask yourself, how can I treat the rete?

The patient will be someone who, even though you have treated every nerve you can think of, still has pain at the very top of their elevation range. Often they will be somebody who carried a heavy bag over that shoulder for years.

Instead of blaming their acromioclavicular joint or sending them in for acromioplasty, treat the rete and see what happens. I do not like direct pressure techniques in general and managed to eliminate most of them, once I realized I was treating nerves, not muscle. This is one of the very few I still use; there just does not seem to be any other way to deal with this problem, because of the peculiarities of the anatomy here. Furthermore, it seems to do the job. Prepare your patient carefully. Fingers are too big to get into the AC notch. The eraser end of a new unsharpened pencil will do the job – you will insert it slowly and carefully, and no further than the eraser itself. It will drag the rete in the direction it seems to need to be dragged, in order for pain to go away and full movement to come back.

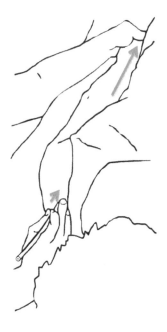

TREATMENT: DIRECT PRESSURE INTO ACROMIOCLAVICULAR
NOTCH WITH PENCIL ERASER

1. Patient can be either prone or supine. Determine which way to have them lie down, by finding their notch first. Some people's AC notch is more posterior, while some are more anterior. Choose which position gives you the most room.

2. Patient's arm is alongside their body. Palm is facing the side of the body.

3. Locate the notch again after the patient has lain down, by tracing the top edge of the clavicle, laterally.

4. Place the eraser end of the pencil at the notch, in line with the arm.

5. Gently grasp patient's hand by the third finger, the axis of the arm.

6. Gently pull the arm longitudinally, while inserting the eraser into the notch.

7. Have the patient take some slow, deep breaths. As they exhale, traction the entire arm through the third finger, and insert the pencil eraser a bit deeper. Do not go deeper than the top end of the eraser. It will feel uncomfortable to them, but if it is the treatment their problem needs, it will also feel oddly good to them at the same time.

8. Stay inside patient's comfort zone. Hold for at least a half-minute.

9. Slowly let go of patient's finger, while easing off the pressure with the pencil.

10. Remove the eraser while pressing down the skin around the notch (as though you were pulling out a long needle).

11. Have the patient stand and recheck elevation, horizontal adduction at shoulder. The annoying pressure pain should feel greatly relieved.

ANTERIOR SHOULDER, ANTERIOR TRUNK

CUTANEOUS NERVES AT FRONT OF SHOULDER:

Ah, here we are at anterior shoulder again, ready to pick up where we left off. Now, however, we have cleared any movement issues or pain or lack of shoulder elevation that may have been stemming from nerves directly underneath, behind, or on top of the shoulder.

Really, though, you can treat what you find in any order you wish. That is your job as a clinician – develop your own way of critically analyzing a situation and deciding what to do, what to examine and/or treat first, then second, and so on. There is no protocol in this work, especially where shoulders are involved.

The embryological story of upper limbs is quite interesting, in my opinion; they are not there right from the start – at first the body plan thinks it is going to be a simple tube with a front end and a tail end. But then a thickening of epidermal tissue forms on each side of the neck – well, not the neck yet, but where the neck will be. All the nerves that will end up in the hand start forming in that thickening, all attached to spinal cord. Then fingers start to form; as excess tissue between them melts away, the hand emerges. Then the arm lengthens behind the hand. And all the nerves and blood vessels in the hand have to lengthen rapidly to stay caught up as the arm forms and grows long. Inside the arm, bone is congealing and muscles are developing. The elongated nerves end up inside tunnels…but I am getting ahead of myself.

Let us look at the front of the shoulder again, and see what can happen right inside the skin organ. At the front of the shoulder is a convergence and possible anastomosing of cutaneous nerve branches from ***supraclavicular nerve*** (C3), ***intercostobrachial anterior branch*** (T2), and ***lateral cutaneous nerve of the arm*** (C5).

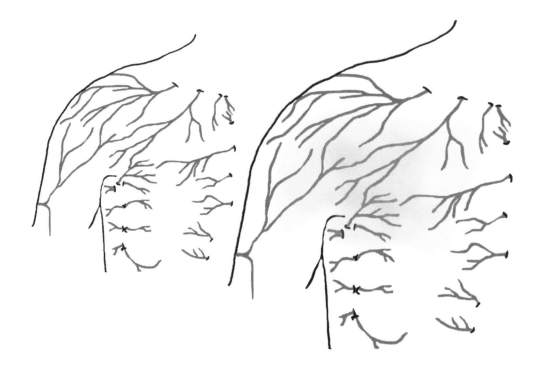

This possibility means (to me at least) that we could ostensibly have a complex neural tunnel problem right inside the skin, not only at the grommet holes where the nerves are exiting into skin organ. Luckily, tenderness usually accompanies pain in front of the shoulder, and tenderness is a useful clue as to whether what we are doing is helping or not helping, during, or has helped, by comparing before/after.

There are a few simple things you can do in this region to move superficial nerves, whether they are anastomosed or not. As always, these are just suggestions – you may improvise as you find necessary.

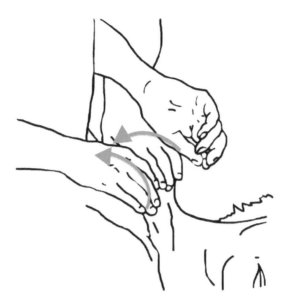

TREATMENT: POSITIONAL RELAXATION APPROACH
COMBINED WITH SKIN STRETCH

1. Patient is sidelying; their back is at the edge of the bed.

2. Stand directly behind patient. You may place a pillow between your body and theirs. Let them lean back against you.

3. Bring your patient's arm into about 45 degrees extension at shoulder, about 60 degrees abduction. Fully support patient's arm under yours, the one closest to patient's head, and hold it with your elbow against your side.

4. Place both hands gently on front of shoulder girdle. Wait for hands to stick to skin.

5. With both hands slowly and gently draw the skin down and around the tendon.

6. Place both thumbs on top of the skin of the large pec major tendon. Wait for them to stick, then draw the skin down and around the pec tendon, toward the axilla. Do not dig in.

7. Hold for about two minutes. Be patient. Feel the patient's physiology adapting to the skin stretch.

8. Carefully let go. Lower arm back down gently to rest on patient's side. Check for tenderness. It should be gone or greatly diminished.

9. Ask patient to stand up, reassess range of movement and how it feels.

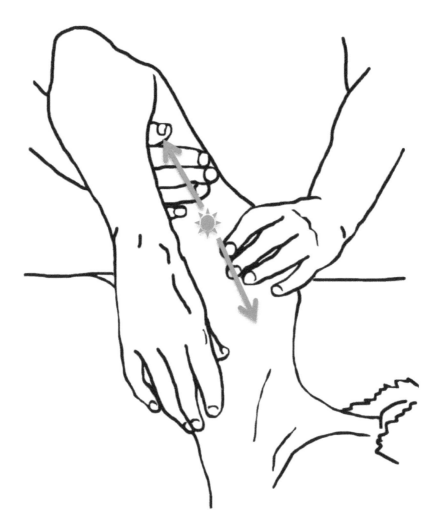

TREATMENT VARIATION: SKIN STRETCH APPROACH

1. Same position as before.

2. Locate sore spot. Place both hands gently on front of shoulder above and below it. Wait for hands to stick to skin.

3. Slowly and gently draw the skin both directions away from it. Hold for two minutes

4. Carefully let go.

5. Ask patient to stand up, reassess range of movement and how it feels.

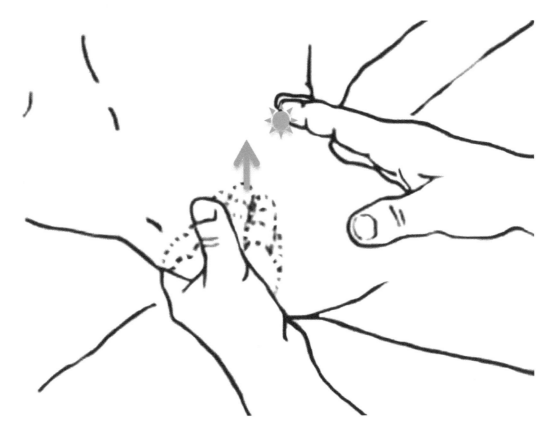

TREATMENT: POSITIONAL RELAXATION APPROACH
COMBINED WITH BALLOONING APPROACH

1. Patient is supine. Therapist sits beside table.
2. Patient's arm rests in about 45 degrees extension, about 30 degrees abduction, on a pillow on top of therapist's lap.
3. Locate sore spot on front of shoulder, monitor only. Place other hand behind shoulder.
4. Press bottom hand upward slowly and firmly against head of humerus, lifting it up toward ceiling slightly.
5. Tender spot will soften and disappear. Hold for about 2 minutes.
6. Slowly remove hands. Ask patient to sit up and explore shoulder movement.

Anterior Cutaneous Nerves of Trunk

We have seen how, as the spinal nerves come round the body, they surface at the back, dorsal rami branching predictably into medial and lateral cutaneous branches, and at the sides of trunk, into anterior and posterior branches. The spinal nerves have one more cutaneous destination – the front of the body.

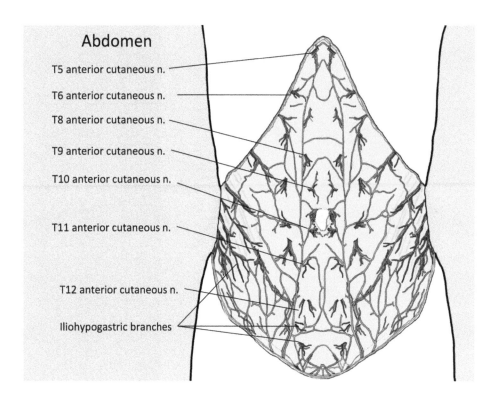

Abdomen

T5 anterior cutaneous n.

T6 anterior cutaneous n.

T8 anterior cutaneous n.

T9 anterior cutaneous n.

T10 anterior cutaneous n.

T11 anterior cutaneous n.

T12 anterior cutaneous n.

Iliohypogastric branches

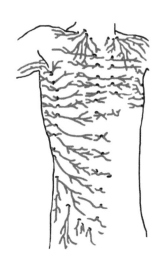
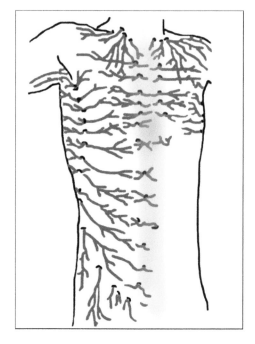

As the body is forming, and the main body tube is enlarging, the spinal nerves are already there, at what will be midline where the two halves of the body wall tube have joined together. Diastasis recti is a condition in which the two sides of the abdominal wall never solidly fused together over the abdomen. Usually the two sides fuse solidly in front, and the cutaneous nerves may overlap the join line somewhat. I have a treatment suggestion for the thoracic nerves, but not for the abdominal cutaneous nerves, not so far anyway. Feel free to design your own. They can become just as entrapped as can any other cutaneous nerve. Non-medical abdominal pain is not common, but it does exist. The front of the body is much less messed up by surgical scarring than in days gone by; however people still have Cesarean sections, which can affect the lowest abdominal cutaneous nerves such as subcostal (T12) and iliohypogastric (L1). The rest of them can become entrapped for other reasons, like hyper-exercising to develop that six-pack. I have had to treat abdominal cutaneous nerves only a few times, though. Treatment of the thoracic anterior cutaneous nerves will be more common.

In the anterior chest, there is a sternum for the surfacing cutaneous nerves to deal with. Here, they have to emerge between ribs, become superficial, then split into their medial and lateral branches. You will need to remember your surface anatomy – the sternum is usually wider than you expect. It's important to find the lateral border of it, because that is where the anterior cutaneous nerve grommet holes are located. And they are *always* tender.

A patient who might benefit from treatment of these nerves will be someone who has had lung or heart problems in the past. They may have had chest tubes. They may be asthmatic. They might mention that they simply cannot take a deep breath. They may appear collapsed in the front, but they might not; they might be just feeling their own interoceptive state. Obviously they can breathe well enough to stay alive, because their diaphragm works and they are in your office, but there is something you can do to help them be able to feel they can expand their chests better – and this is, help them to notice their sore spots better.

Normally I avoid direct pressure on sore spots; however, this area is pretty special, and most of the time people have no idea how sore these spots really are. You do not have to press hard on them to activate nociceptive processing in them. You can think about it as letting the brain in on the fact they are really sore, and activating all the power it has to kick up opioid production immediately in a region so important for life processes and homeostasis of its organism. One hand is in front, and the other hand is behind, on a sore spot near the spine, on the same segmental level, where the dorsal rami emerge between ribs at the back. (Even though you are not doing anything to treat ribs, you need to be able to find and *feel* ribs, and spinous processes, in order to know what level you are on back there - you will need to remember your surface anatomy! You might want to practice this on a skeletal model first to review hand placement.)

The first anterior cutaneous nerve is behind the clavicle and emerges in the sternal notch. You will only need to be concerned here with the anterior cutaneous exit points for spinal nerves T2 through T6, because these nerves have the sternum, and therefore fibro osseous tunnels, to contend with.

After T6 or 7, rib attachments in front become cartilaginous and descend laterally and obliquely, and the rest of the anterior cutaneous nerves, 7 through 12, come out down the front of the abdominal wall.

INDICATION: THE FEELING OF NOT BEING ABLE TO BREATHE DEEPLY OR EXPAND CHEST FULLY, POOR EXCURSION OF RIBCAGE, RIBCAGE STIFFNESS

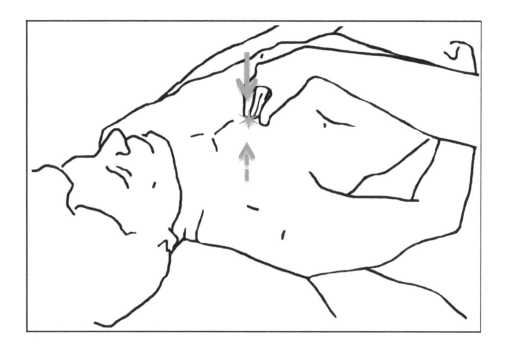

TREATMENT: COUNTER IRRITATION APPROACH

1. Patient is supine, legs comfortably supported over a bolster.
2. Slide one hand behind back, just off spinous process – locate a tender spot (medial branch of dorsal cutaneous nerve), between two ribs. Press on one of the ribs at the back with some convenient finger, and feel with the other hand which rib has moved, so you can be oriented to the appropriate level in front.
3. With other hand, locate tender spot between ribs, just off lateral border of sternum, at corresponding level where anterior cutaneous nerve emerges.
4. Press with single fingertip from above and below, carefully. These will be tender.
5. Hold for about 30 seconds. Tenderness will rapidly decrease.
6. Move to next level. Repeat.
7. When one side of the ribcage is completed, ask patient to stand and check deep breathing. Patient will feel much increased sense of space and ability to inhale on that side compared to the other.
8. Repeat other side.

NERVES OF THE ARM, ELBOW, FOREARM AND HAND

As mentioned earlier, long nerves of the arm (with the exception of the musculocutaneous nerve) start out in embryological life embedded inside the hand; as the arm lengthens out behind the hand, they grow longer and end up enclosed in fibro osseous tunnels at the wrist and elbow, where the bony skeleton is wider and soft tissue more scarce.

As we approach the distal ends of limbs, the brain devotes more cortical real estate to the maps it has of the skin of those areas. Put another way, there are much, much smaller receptive fields and there is greater sensory discrimination (than compared to, for example, skin on the back), especially of the glabrous skin of the hand, where two of the long nerves terminate cutaneously. However, the entire arm is *loaded* with cutaneous nerves, which, collectively;

1. Are unique branches from the brachial plexus, or from T2, such as the ones serving the medial aspect of the arm,
2. Are branches that have split off the long nerves higher up, such as the cutaneous nerves on the back and lateral side of the upper arm from the radial nerve,
3. Represent a unique sensory and autonomic fascicle of a nerve that started out being primarily motor, such as the musculocutaneous nerve that innervates coracobrachialis and elbow flexors, then becomes lateral cutaneous nerve of the forearm.

CUTANEOUS NERVES OF THE ARM

Let us take a look at cutaneous nerves of the arm.

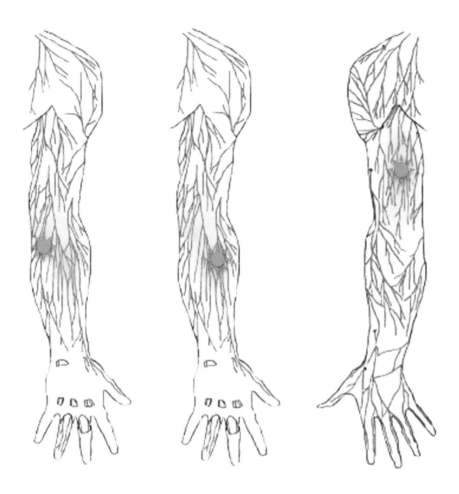

Cutaneous nerves are everywhere, and they can hurt anywhere.

First we will look at how they might be treated individually, based on finding and addressing tender points. The example is for a tender point at the back of the arm, but this approach may be applied to sore spots anywhere, front, back, arm or forearm.

I like to treat arms in a modified quadruped position, which means, with the arm hanging freely; I like it for three reasons. First, I can make gravity my helper. Second, it is easy to reach anywhere on the arm and use a balloon approach. Third, I think there might be some deeply buried neurological advantage, in that during most of evolutionary time, peripheral nerves in quadrupeds existed at this angle to the rest of the body; so I think it may create more slack for them and for the vasculature that supplies them, especially at the shoulder. Anything to shorten and widen the overall neural container for the entire neurovascular peripheral tree.

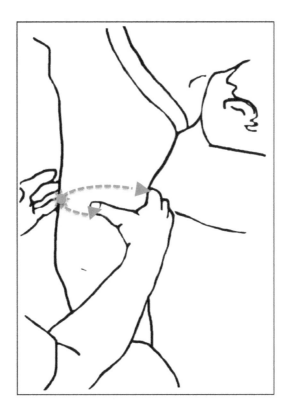

TREATMENT: SKIN STRETCH APPROACH COMBINED WITH BALLOONING

1. Patient is prone, arm hanging freely in 90 degrees of shoulder flexion, or resting on therapist's knee – whichever is more comfortable for the patient.
2. Find tender point behind arm. Place other hand gently on front of arm, carefully pull skin layer forward, in a gentle pinch grasp
3. Tender spot will soften, tenderness will disappear
4. Hold for 2 minutes. Slowly let go.
5. Ask patient to sit up and move arm

A group approach to these nerves can also be tried. Especially for someone who has been in a lot of pain for a long time, a global approach can feel luxuriously relaxing. I have noticed over the years, somewhat of a directional preference, as depicted below. S-shaped stretches of skin feel particularly pleasant; the interoceptive impression is that the arm is kinesthetically lengthening. They can be applied to skin above and below the elbow, as indicated by arrows in the diagram below, with the patient in prone position, with arm dangling freely.

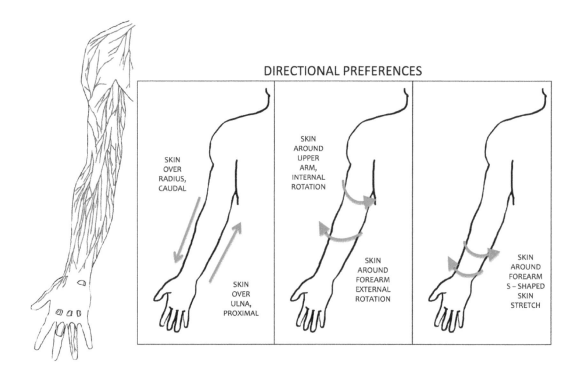

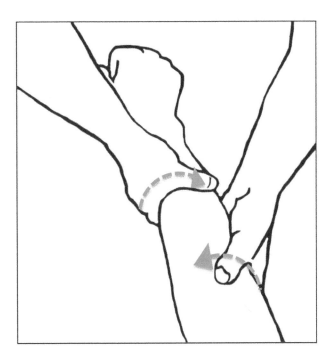

TREATMENT: S-SHAPED SKIN STRETCH APPROACH

1. Patient and arm can be in any position, well supported

2. Grasp skin of forearm gently with both hands. Wait for hands to stick to skin.

3. Gently and slowly twist skin layer opposite directions in large S-shape. Hold for at least 2 minutes. Therapist will feel a great deal of motion intrinsic to forearm, sometimes movement of arm itself. Slowly let go.

4. Ask patient to move forearm, hand, wrist, and report.

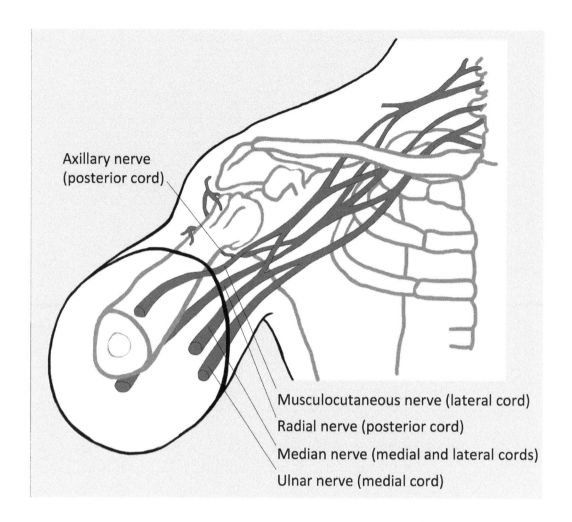

Axillary nerve
(posterior cord)

Musculocutaneous nerve (lateral cord)

Radial nerve (posterior cord)

Median nerve (medial and lateral cords)

Ulnar nerve (medial cord)

Here are some images that show their pathways and what they innervate along the way.

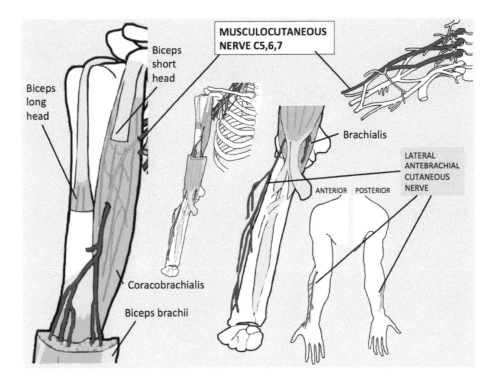

Musculocutaneous

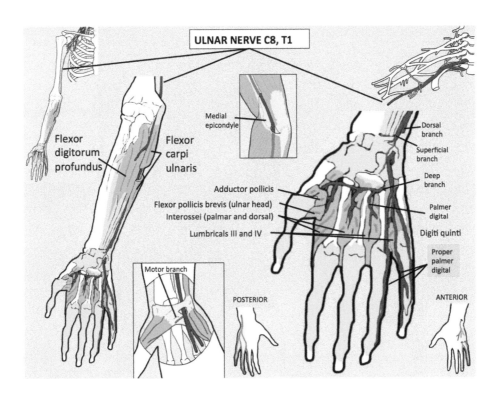

Ulnar

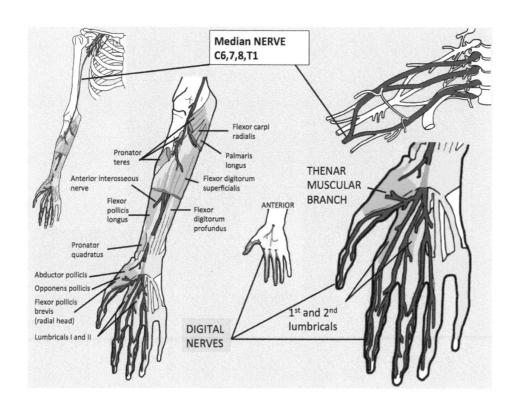

Median

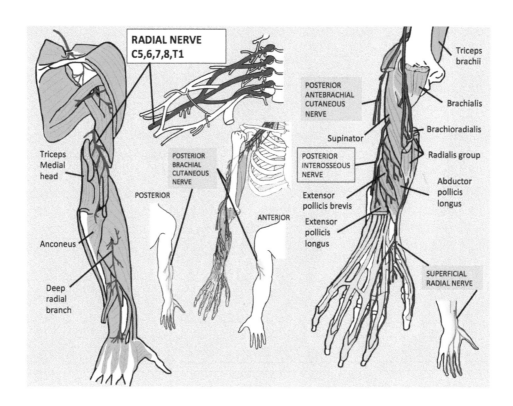

Radial

DermoNeuroModulating | Diane Jacobs

You do not have to think much about the muscles innervated by these long nerves unless you come across a rare patient in whom one or more muscles in hand or arm are paralyzed. Instead, we are confronted mostly by people who have pain issues anywhere in arm or hand. So, think about nerves themselves instead. Why? Because pain is a nervous system phenomenon, not a muscle phenomenon.

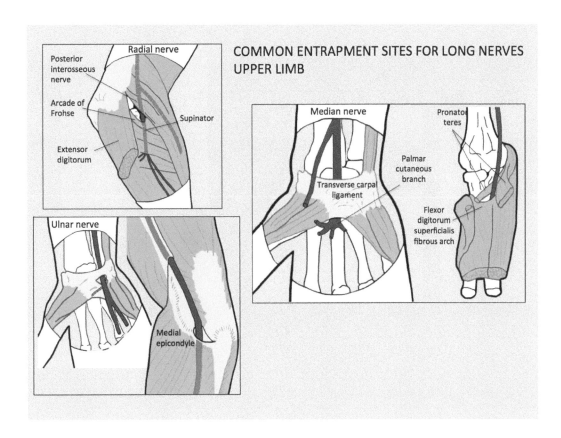

Common entrapment sites

Where long bones meet, they flare. Tendons attach. Ranges of movement become large and hugely angled. Where long bones attach to hands, they attach to a bunch of tiny bones without much meat, but with a *lot* of tendons over them, held down by thick unforgiving ligaments. These are danger zones for nerves because not only do their tunnels narrow but also they have to slide against unforgiving bone.

Now, about those entrapment sites at elbow and wrist: it may seem counterintuitive; *however,* ballooning techniques, which appear to pull the nerve even closer to the bone, may actually *widen or spread the neural tunnel* around the nerve, or at least distort it enough, for a little while, so that the nerve may be able to adjust and normalize its local physiology. Allow tenderness, and decrease thereof, to be your guide. You can also track palpable softening of the tissue, and let that be an added guide.

INDICATION: POINT TENDERNESS AT ELBOW, PAIN ON MOVEMENT, POSSIBLE DISTAL PARESTHESIA IN ULNAR DISTRIBUTION

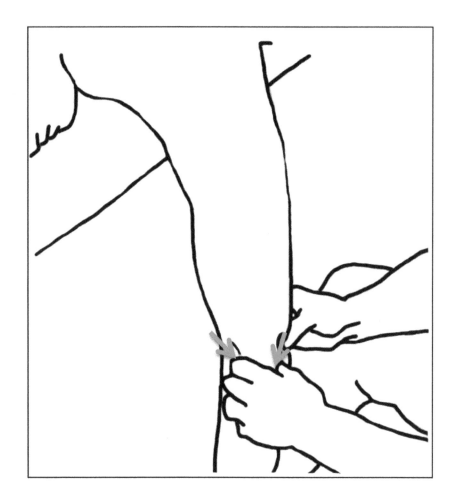

TREATMENT: SKIN STRETCH APPROACH USING BALLOON TECHNIQUE

1. Arm hangs freely in 90 degrees of flexion with patient prone.
2. Find point tenderness medial side of elbow. Use other hand to perform a gentle grasp technique; pull skin away from sore side around to opposite side.
3. Tenderness will decrease and point will soften. Hold for 2 minutes.
4. Let go slowly, ask patient to sit up and move elbow, reassess pain on movement.

NOTE: Same technique can be used for any neural tunnel at elbow at elbow.

- If you want to decompress the neural tunnel for radial nerve, balloon at the medial side of elbow.

- If you want to decompress the neural tunnel for the median nerve, balloon at the back of the elbow.

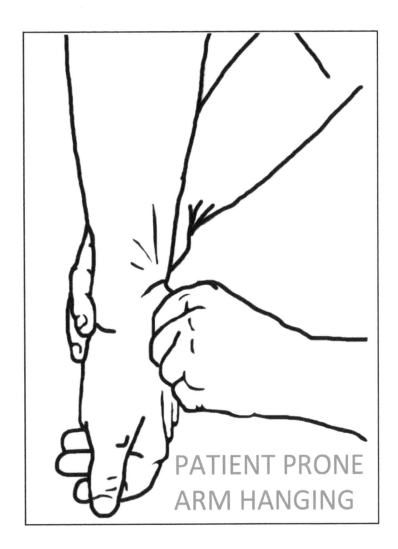

PATIENT PRONE
ARM HANGING

TREATMENT: SKIN STRETCH APPROACH USING BALLOON TECHNIQUE

1. Patient may be in any position. Support arm fully. Locate a tender point in anterior hand or wrist, and monitor.

2. With other hand slowly and gently grasp skin on back of hand, and by stages, pull it tight, around entire hand. Twist it a little, clockwise or anticlockwise, whichever way seems to achieve the most reduction in tenderness and increase in softening. Hold for about 2 minutes, longer if necessary.

3. Let go slowly.

4. Remove your hands, ask patient to move hand, reassess range and comfort level.

5. You might want to teach patients how to do this by themselves, several times a day, to relieve the discomfort of their job, if their job puts undue strain on their wrist.

NERVES OF THE HAND

Cutaneous nerves of the hand are subject to a lot of variation in how they self-organize, anastomose, etc.

CUTANEOUS NERVES OF HANDS

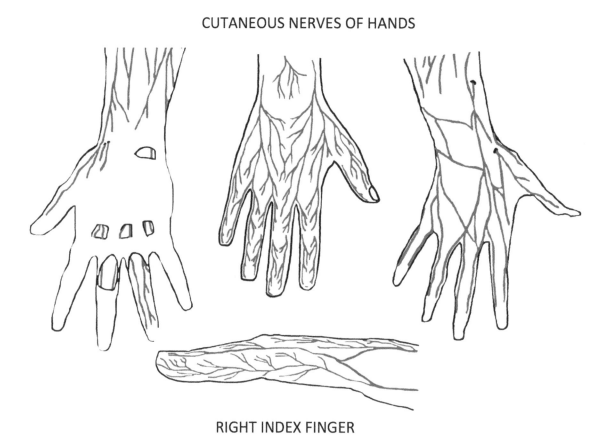

RIGHT INDEX FINGER

Remember that hands, particularly the glabrous surface, have exquisite sensory discriminative capacity. They also have a great deal of small receptive field nociceptive capacity, as we learn when we sustain a paper cut!

Nothing feels quite as delicious as good handling does, when applied to pain felt in a hand. There are so many bones, so little meat, so many neural tunnels, so much three-dimensional movement to be explored.

There are some very basic movements of the hand, and directional preferences of the skin organ I have noticed, depicted below.

DIRECTIONAL PREFERENCES

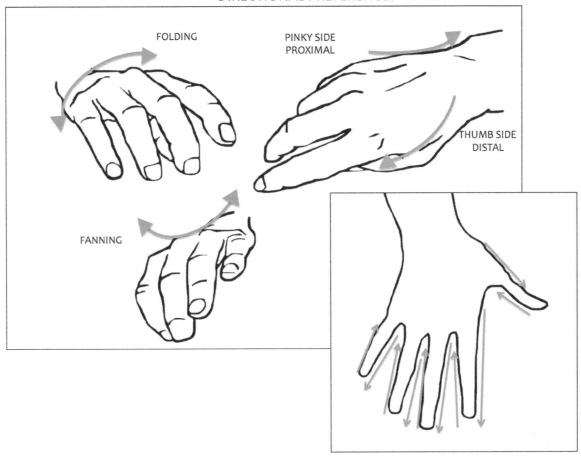

FOLDING

PINKY SIDE PROXIMAL

THUMB SIDE DISTAL

FANNING

Some treatment suggestions follow, but really, you can just relax and let your hands themselves be your guide.

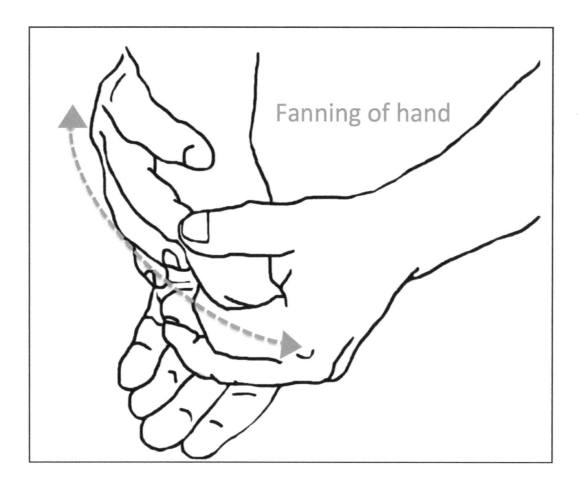

Fanning of hand

TREATMENT: SKIN STRETCH APPROACH

1. Patient may be in any position. Support arm fully.

2. Slowly and gently grasp entire hand. By stages, pull it open. Hold for 2 minutes. Let go slowly.

3. Remove your hands, ask patient to move hand, reassess range and comfort level

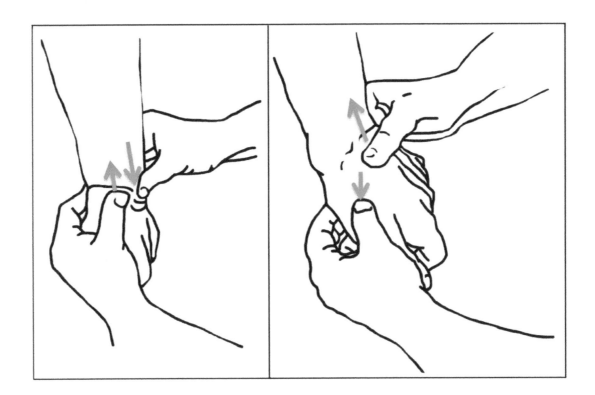

INDICATION: HAND PAIN, STIFFNESS

TREATMENT: SKIN STRETCH APPROACH

1. Patient may be in any position. Support arm fully.

2. Slowly and gently grasp entire hand. By stages, move skin gently in directions shown. Hold for 2 minutes. Let go slowly.

3. Remove your hands, ask patient to move hand, reassess range and comfort level

4. If the first direction does not result in completely decreased discomfort, try another.

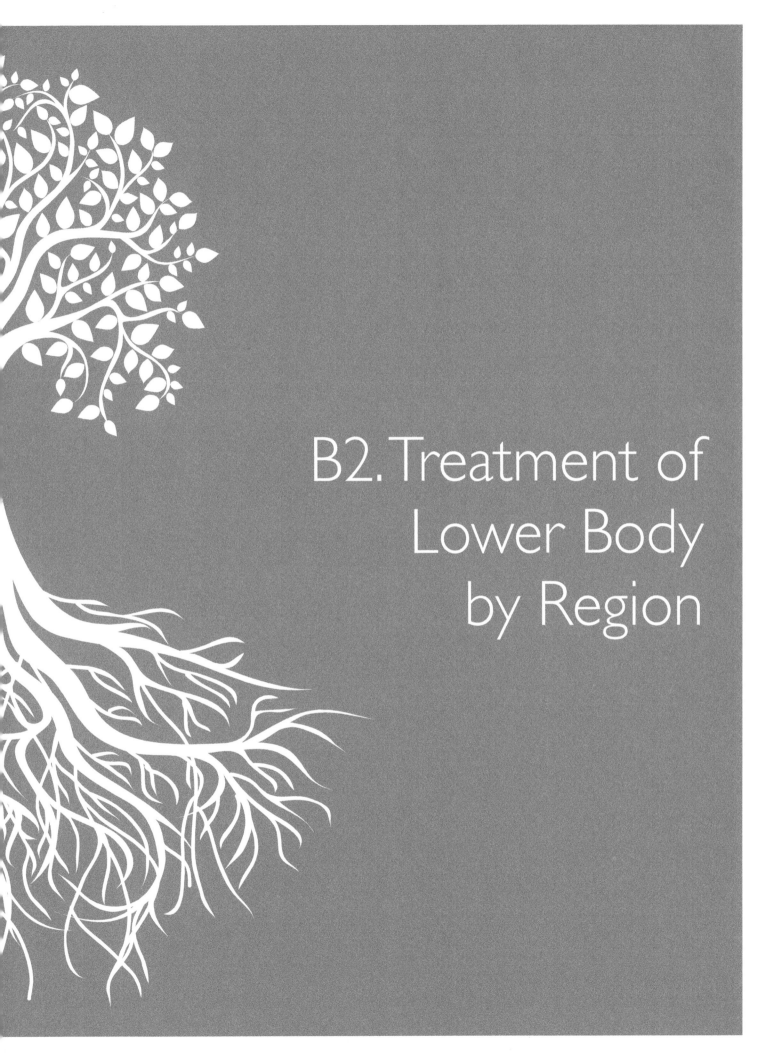

B2. Treatment of Lower Body by Region

THE BACK

DORSAL RAMI

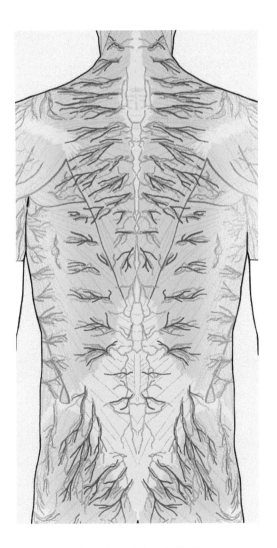

Dorsal rami of entire back

Here we are, back to posterior trunk, once again dealing with dorsal rami. We left off at about the bottom of the rib cage, or T12 level.

Before we deal with the lower back, let us step back for a wide view of the whole back, and some simple treatment ideas we can use for cutaneous nerves anywhere in the back.

In an effort to put the entire neural tree into a quadruped position, one can choose a flexed sidelying position. If you want to treat prone, that is fine. However, people might be more comfortable with their hips flexed a little; I use foam wedges or a pillow. I also have a headrest that tilts down to flex the spinal cord slightly. The objective is to shorten and widen the whole body, which forms a neural container for the entire neural tree, that 72-kilometer, 45-mile bunch of peripheral nerves we have. Remember that the back does not have very good sensory discrimination. Receptive fields are huge. Stretching skin, whether over small areas or over large swathes of back, feels really good. It usually results in large increases in effortless range of motion. Not bad for something so global and generic.

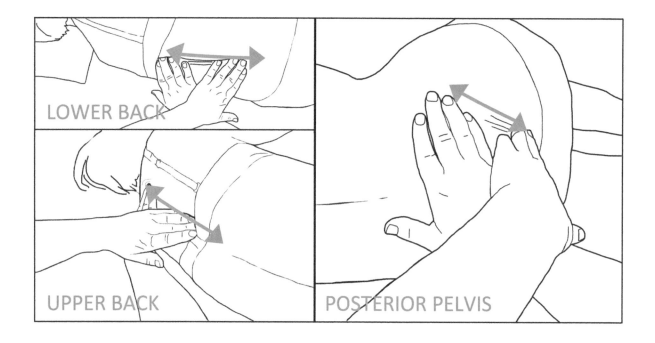

Patient is in left sidelying. One can stretch skin in small zones anywhere dorsal rami exist. The diagram shows the stretch being parallel to the spinous processes, and to edge of sacrum. But really, it can be done anywhere in any direction.

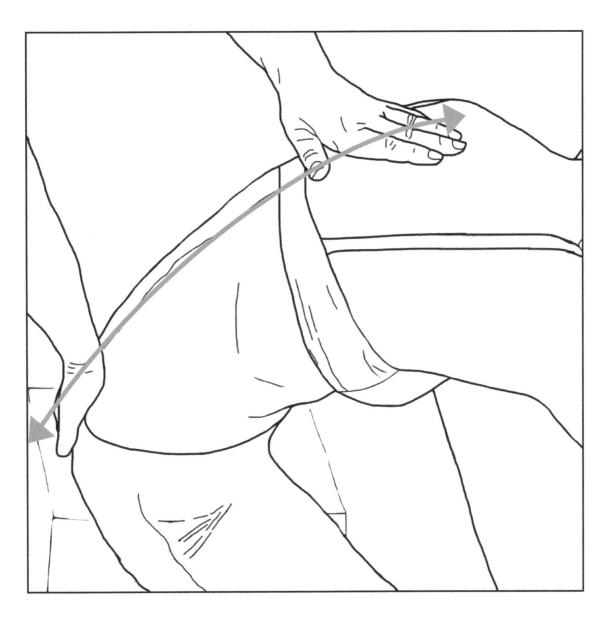

Skin stretch in seated position, entire length of spine. Added pressure over sacrum, slowly loaded in, feels really good to most people.

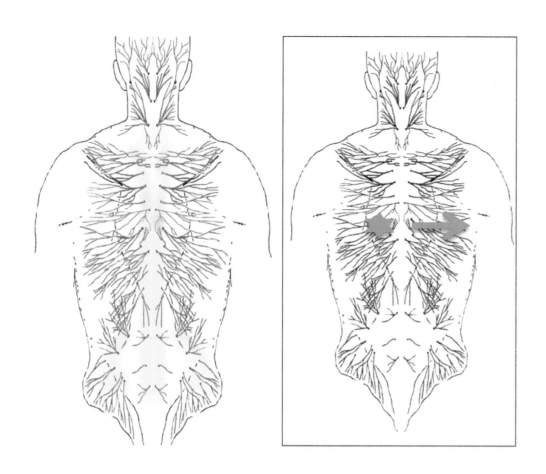

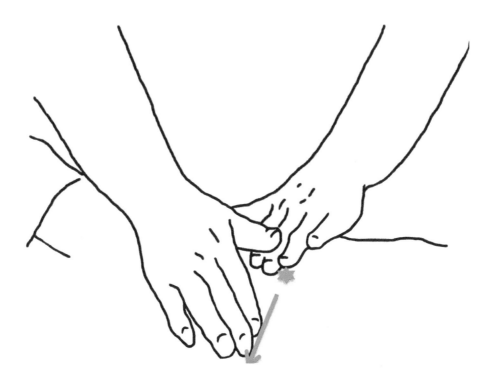

TREATMENT: SKIN STRETCH APPROACH, ACROSS
SPINE TARGETING MEDIAL BRANCH

1. Patient is prone.
2. Locate sore spot – monitor it with one hand
3. Draw skin away from it, using other hand, across midline
4. Wait for softening, and then hold for a few minutes. You may twist the skin slightly clockwise or counterclockwise if that improves the softening.
5. Let go slowly.
6. Ask patient to stand, move about, and perform range of movement testing, to confirm/ consolidate improvement.

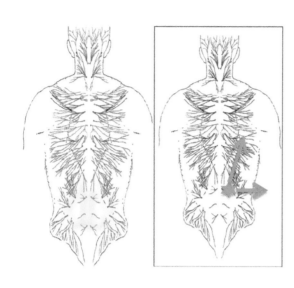 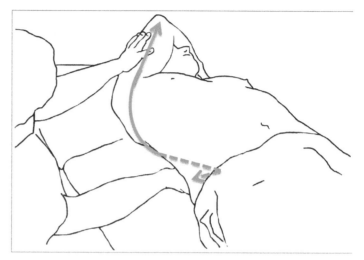

TREATMENT: SKIN STRETCH APPROACH TARGETING LATERAL BRANCH

1. Patient is supine, legs resting comfortably over a bolster.

2. Slide one hand in behind patient - locate sore spot – monitor it with one hand.

3. With the other hand, elevate arm on same side. Place free hand on the back of the arm. Wait until your hand sticks to the patient's skin.

4. Carefully drag the skin on the back of patient's arm toward their elbow. Under your monitoring hand you should be able to feel the skin move a little, and suddenly, some softening will occur, and tenderness will disappear.

5. Hold everything in that position for a few minutes. With monitoring hand, pull the skin on the patient's back, laterally, away from spine, if that improves the softening.

6. Let go slowly.

7. Ask patient to stand, move about, and perform range of movement testing, to confirm/consolidate improvement.

What do you do if there is a lot of pain of recent onset, and your patient walks in very uncomfortable with any specific movement? This is unlikely to be something that will resolve with superficial treatment only. It likely will not be entrapment of only a superficial part of a dorsal ramus. It may be an entrapped dorsal ramus at a deeper level, or maybe even a ventral ramus. No way to know for sure. However, here are some innocuous, time-tested, and very boiled-down approaches one can try. The patient will retain locus of control.

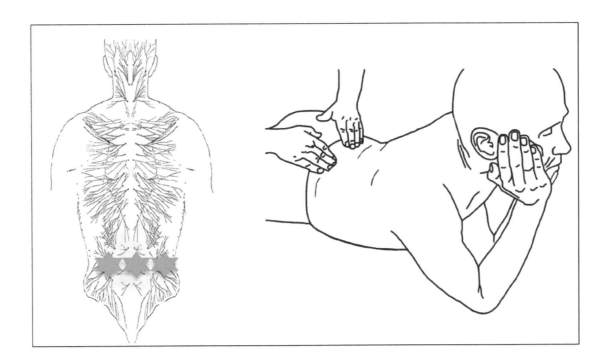

ASSESSMENT:

1. Ask your patient to lie prone, up on their elbows with their chin supported by their hands. Make sure the forearms are vertical.

2. On assessment with gravity eliminated as much as possible, one can see that while one side of the low back can easily drop down into extended position, and tolerate a bit of pressure, but the other side cannot.

3. Since most of us are right handed, usually the side that cannot drop down will be the left side, but not 100% of the time.

4. If you are still not sure which side needs treated, for example, if they *both* look like they cannot extend, you can always go ahead and treat both sides.

5. In this example the patient is a typical right-handed individual, whose low back on the left side cannot drop easily down into extension. If your patient is left-handed, it may be the right side of their low back that cannot fully extend.

INDICATION: BACK PAIN MOSTLY ON ONE SIDE, USUALLY RECENT ONSET,
WITH INABILITY TO BEND BACKWARD ON ONE SIDE IN PRONE

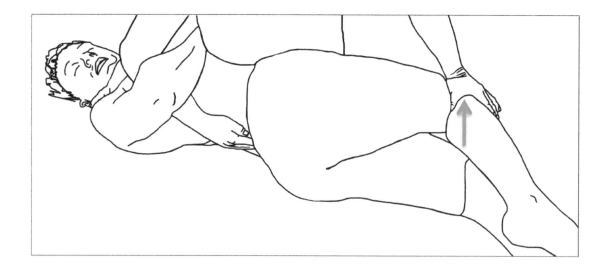

TREATMENT: POSITIONAL RELAXATION APPROACH
COMBINED WITH CONTRACT-RELAX APPROACH

1. Patient lies on table in side lying, restricted side down.

2. Ask patient to come right to the edge of the table. Put your fist on the edge of the table with your arm vertical, and ask the patient to come right up against your arm. Tell them you will not let them fall off the bed.

3. Stand sideways, facing the patient's head, and block patient's body with your hip; monitor their back with one hand, use the other to draw their bottom arm forward (which will roll their upper trunk toward supine).

4. Turn yourself around to support patient with your other hip, and change hands.

5. Ask patient to link their upper arm with yours, as though they were square dancing. Being able to hang on to your arm will give them reassurance that they will not fall off the bed.

6. With your free hand, extend their bottom leg. Ask them to help you a little. The bottom leg needs to be fully extended and parallel to the edge of the bed.

7. Fold the top leg carefully into flexion. Monitor low back, and fold upper leg up until you feel slight movement in their back, under your monitoring hand. That will be far enough. They will now be rotated in this sidelying horizontal position. Their knee should be well over the edge of the bed.

8. Place your hand on top of the top knee. But do not push down! You are not going to crack their back. Verbally state that to the patient.

DermoNeuroModulating | Diane Jacobs

9. Instead, ask patient to press top knee gently up against your hand, hold for 5-10 seconds, and then relax.

10. Take the top leg into a bit more flexion and roll the upper body of the patient into a little more rotation toward supine to take up any slack that has been created.

11. Repeat the process from step 8-10, two more times.

12. Allow patient to roll completely onto their back for a moment. Then have them roll over prone, and reassess. Both sides of the back should now be able to drop down easily.

13. Ask patient to get up and walk around, try bending over, side-bending etc. They will usually be able to move much easier than they could before.

An identical scenario: your patient walks in very uncomfortable with any specific movement.

So, you look at their extension and it seems fine on both sides, looks symmetric.

Now what?

Well, check their flexion to see if *it* looks bilaterally symmetric.

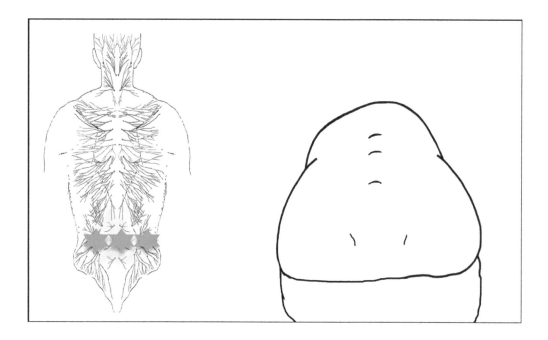

ASSESSMENT:

Ask the patient to sit down and bend forward between their knees, wide apart. They usually can, slowly.

You will usually see that one side is able to bend forward a lot easier than the other side – the restricted side will appear humped up more.

Furthermore, usually these people will usually be able to move easier with range of movement testing into extension and sidebend in standing, and have pain-restricted movement mainly on forward flexion in standing.

Again, most of the restricted flexion problems seem to be mainly on one side, usually the *right* side. Again, I am pretty sure that this relates to which hand is dominant.

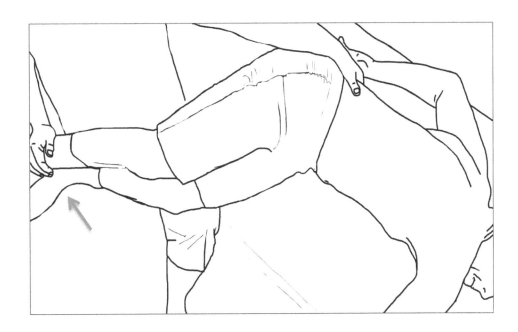

TREATMENT: POSITIONAL RELAXATION APPROACH
COMBINED WITH CONTRACT-RELAX APPROACH

1. It is easiest to just demonstrate the position you want the patient to assume, rather than trying to talk them through it.

2. Patient lies on table with upper trunk prone, lower trunk rotated, "restricted" side up. Ask them to move their upper body closer to the opposite side of the bed, and lower body closer to the side where you are standing. Their hips and knees are together and both are flexed slightly.

3. You will sit on the table with both the patient's legs over your lap. Just lift them up, and slide in underneath them. One foot may need to be up on a short stool to balance the legs comfortably across thigh. You can now control patient's trunk flexion, side bend, and rotation, through their lower limbs.

4. Bend patient's lower body into slightly more flexion and/or side bend, to find an optimal place to start. One hand monitors the patient's back while other rests on patient's feet, ankles together.

5. Ask patient to press *both* ankles, *gently*, up against your hand, hold for 5-10 seconds, and then relax. The smallest pressure they can manage will be perfectly adequate.

6. Find the next position for patient's legs to rest in, by monitoring the back with one hand, and moving yourself together with patient's legs to take up any new slack that has presented itself.

7. Repeat the contract-relax process twice more.

SUPERIOR CLUNEAL NERVES

There are long (very long!) dorsal rami that disseminate downward and obliquely within the back, and emerge at the rim of the pelvis to supply the skin over the buttocks. They are called the **superior cluneal nerves**. They come from L1, 2, and 3.

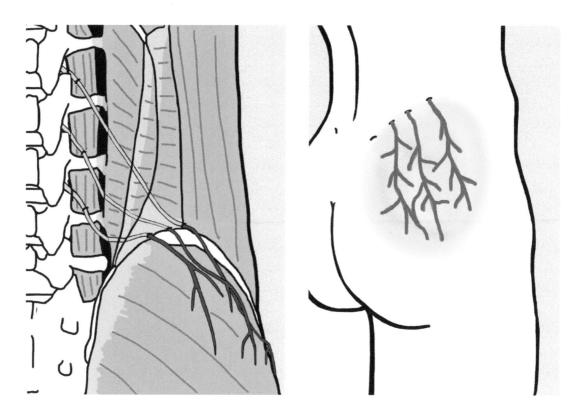

Right at the upper edge of the posterior pelvis, they can become entrapped in their fibro osseous tunnels. They can become *so* entrapped that large tender bumps form at the grommet holes. These can occur in anyone, but seem to be the most common in people who are sedentary, in people who wear tool belts, in truckers who have not learned to take out their wallet from their back pocket. They are associated with nagging dull constant backache.

Many patients may have no apparent movement dysfunction, yet still describe longstanding, nagging toothache kind of pain with point tenderness, in the low back or lower, over the sacrum, or off to the side of it. This sort of presentation may represent entrapment of some small branch of a superior or medial cluneal nerve, and may benefit from a positional relaxation approach. The leg is taken into extension to shorten and widen the neural tunnel of a superior cluneal nerve. 'Twizzle' is added, in an attempt to torque nerve and neural tunnel against each other.

INDICATION: DULL CONSTANT NAGGING BACKACHE WITH LARGE PALPABLE TENDER NODULES ALONG POSTERIOR RIM OF PELVIS

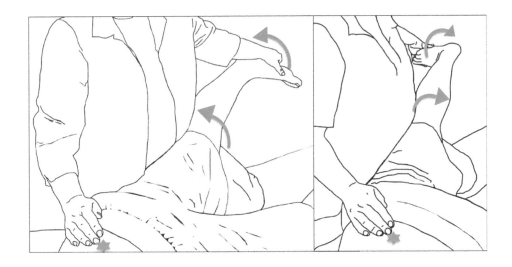

TREATMENT: POSITIONAL RELAXATION APPROACH WITH 'TWIZZLE' THROUGH THE FOOT

1. Patient is prone.

2. Sore spot is located and monitored.

3. Lift patient's leg up onto your knee.

4. Grasp their foot comfortably with the other hand.

5. Torque their foot, slowly and carefully, into either internal or external rotation, which ever way works best for that individual, until tenderness disappears.

6. Then hold their foot and leg in that position for about 2 minutes.

7. Let go slowly.

8. Ask patient to stand, move about, perform range of movement testing, to confirm/consolidate improvement

You could try any of the skin stretch approaches previously described, as well. Be inventive - the world of manual therapy is yours to add to.

Once in awhile you will get a patient who has nagging dull constant back pain higher up.

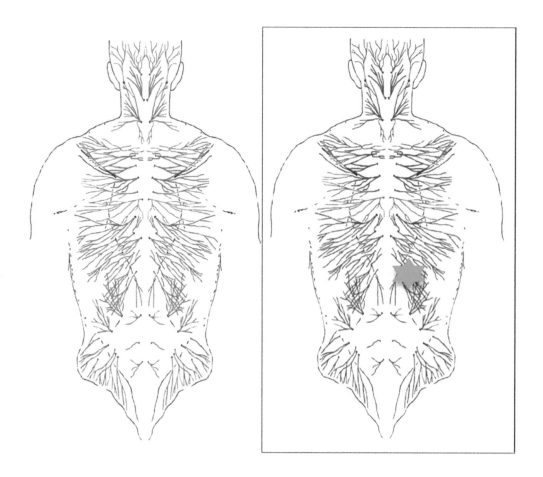

When you assess them, they will have pretty good side bend one way but not the other. When you palpate them in prone, they will have an area of tightness at or very near their thoracolumbar junction, in the zone from about L1 to L3. It seems this tightness will just not disappear, no matter what you try. Everyone tends to blame quadratus lumborum for this, but I insist it is not a muscle causing the problem, only reacting to the problem. What is the problem? Some neural entrapment of some kind, with the added complication of floating ribs that up space.

So, here is one more thing you can try: lateral ribcage squishing.

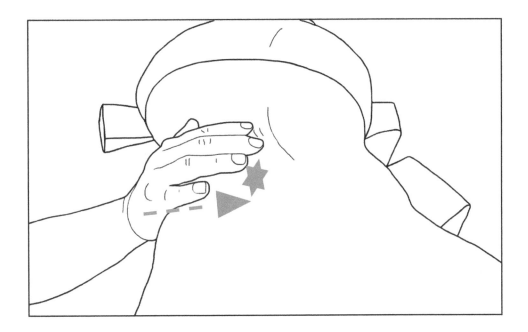

TREATMENT: POSITIONAL RELAXATION APPROACH COMBINED WITH DIRECT PRESSURE AGAINST SIDE OF RIBCAGE

1. Patient is prone.

2. Place body into side flexion, convex to side to be treated (like the letter "C"). Bank up the concave side, by placing a wedge under ribcage

3. Place a wedge under each side of pelvis, to block sliding.

4. Locate sore spot – it may be monitored with one hand.

5. Place other hand on side of ribcage. It is good to use a thick piece of foam to spread out the force and make the process more comfortable.

6. Carefully load in pressure, from the side, directly toward middle of body. Add a bit of torque if necessary, and if desirable.

7. If your patient is large and you are small or if your hand is small, you may need to use your own sternum and body weight.

8. Wait for softening and then hold for a few minutes.

9. Let go slowly.

10. Ask patient to stand, move about, and perform range of movement testing, to confirm/consolidate improvement.

POSTERIOR PELVIS

POSTERIOR PELVIS

Cutaneous dorsal rami from L 4 and 5 exist, but are quite short, and only supply that little area right over the levels from which they emerge. Most of the spinal nerves from L4 and 5 go into making up the huge sciatic nerve, which is ventral, and will be discussed later. All skin organ over the superior aspect of buttocks and over sacrum, is supplied by superior cluneal nerves from L1,2, and 3, and medial cluneal nerves from S1, 2, and 3.

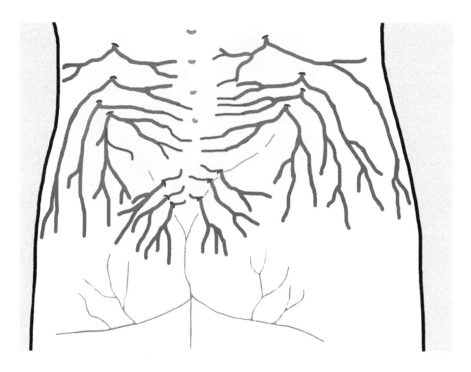

Superior and medial cluneal nerves

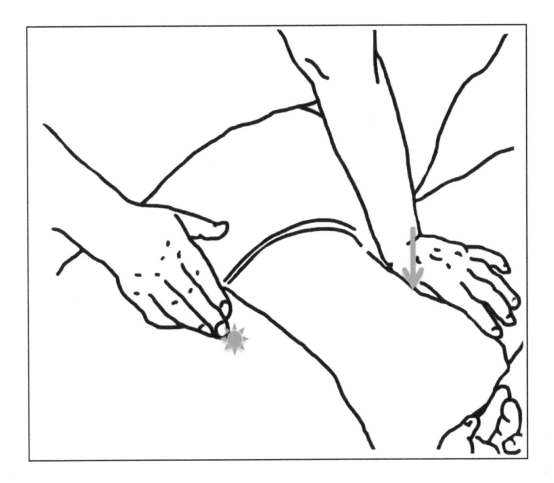

NOTE: There may be several tender spots within a small area. Be patient

1. Locate tender point anywhere in low back below posterior rim of pelvis, monitor with one hand

2. Place heel other hand directly over posterior side of trochanter. Wait for hand to stick to skin

3. Gradually press skin over trochanter, and trochanter itself, directly downward. Cutaneous nerves will be pulled through their tunnels over pelvic rim. Tender spot will soften and disappear.

4. Hold 2 minutes

5. Slowly let go. Ask patient to stand and move, to confirm/consolidate improvement.

MEDIAL CLUNEAL NERVES

Medial cluneal nerves are the cutaneous dorsal rami of S1, 2 and 3, and emerge from holes in the sacrum at S1, 2 and 3.

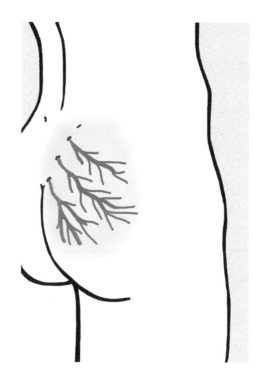

They not only have to make it out through osseous holes in the sacrum, they have to make it through a lot of very tough ligamentous material along the way, where long back muscles are attached to the top surface of the sacrum, in layers. From most deepest to most superficial, layers include the posterior sacroiliac ligament, and attachments of:

1. multifidus
2. longissimus thoracis
3. iliocostalis lumborum
4. latissimus dorsi

The sacroiliac joints are often blamed for pain in this neighbourhood, but, like everything else structural, they are usually completely innocent. One can first treat for any possible neural tunnel distress in the vicinity, superficially, by doing skin stretching, and see what happens. Usually pain goes away and effortless, full movement returns.

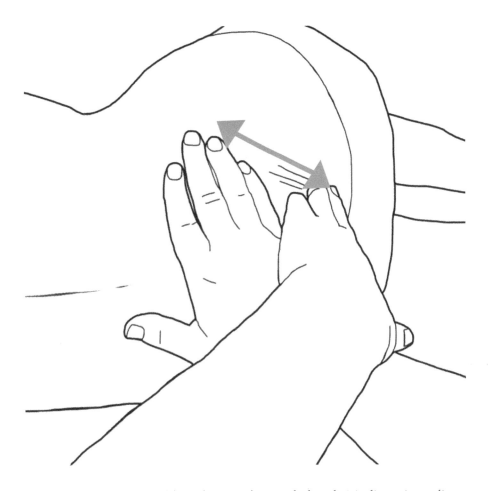

Image shows patient in sidelying; however, skin stretch along the joint line, or in any direction along or across sacrum, may be applied in prone lying as well

TREATMENT: SKIN STRETCH APPROACH

1. Patient is in sidelying.

2. Using both hands, carefully make contact with skin along the diagonal lateral border of the sacrum.

3. Draw hands apart, applying slight stretch to skin between hands.

4. Hold for about two minutes.

5. Let go slowly.

6. Palpate for any tenderness there may be in the vicinity, and stretch skin in any creative ways that you find may reduce it.

DEEP MOTOR NERVES IN THE REGION

There are deeper nerves in the buttock region, of course. Gluteal nerves emerge through the sciatic notch to innervate the gluteal muscles from beneath. Other deep neural branches innervate other deep hip muscles.

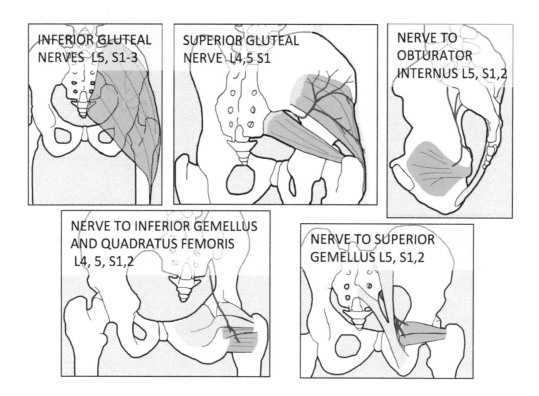

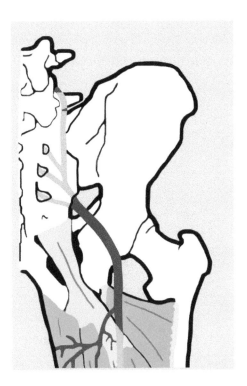

The sciatic nerve emerges deep in this region, with its occasionally problematic relationship with piriformis muscle, which comprises part of its neural tunnel. These nerves are all from ventral roots of the lumbosacral plexus. They do not have cutaneous branches in this zone. However, it is possible to treat them as a group by altering the tunnels through which they must emerge.

The classic patient is someone who has had a deep and annoying pain in the buttock for any length of time, sometimes for years or even decades. They have tried lying on a golf ball, have had people press elbows into their flesh, etc., but still, they cannot seem to get rid of this pain. They may have reduced hip drop on that side. These individuals may benefit greatly from a positional relaxation approach combined with an added "twizzle."

INDICATION: PAIN IN THE BUTTOCK OF ANY DURATION; POSSIBLY,
DULL PAIN ON STRAIGHT LEG RAISE; POSSIBLE REDUCED HIP DROP

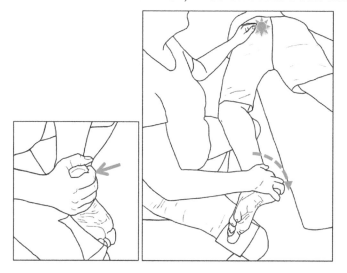

TREATMENT: POSITIONAL RELAXATION APPROACH
COMBINED WITH 'TWIZZLING' THROUGH THE FOOT

1. Patient is prone.

2. Bring their leg off side of bed, into about 45 degrees flexion/abduction at hip, 45 degrees
    knee flexion, resting on seated therapist's knee.

3. Keep lower leg parallel to the edge of the bed.

4. With one hand, find the tender point. It will be deep. You may not be able to feel anything,
    so ask the patient to let you know when you are on it.

5. With other hand, hook lateral side of patient's foot against your knee and carefully pull their
    heel toward you, taking the whole foot into inversion and lower leg into internal rotation.
    Check in with the patient to make sure their ankle is comfortable throughout the process.
    Nothing in the buttock will improve if the patient has to deal with pain in their foot.

6. Tenderness will disappear.

7. Hold at least 2 minutes, and then slowly let go. Ask patient to stand

8. Check for improvement in movement.

TREATMENT VARIATION (REVERSE TWIZZLE):

1. Place patient in the exact same set-up.

2. Place *medial* border of their foot upon your knee. Push heel away, into increased abduction/
    eversion of foot, and external rotation of lower leg.

We are going to skip over inferior cluneal nerves and coccygeal plexus at this time, and consider
them later when we discuss treatment for nerves of the pelvic floor.

LATERAL PELVIS AND LATERAL HIP

LATERAL BRANCH OF ILIOHYPOGASTRIC NERVE

As we come around the side of the pelvis, another long nerve of significance that drapes down through the body wall to emerge cutaneously, over the lateral edge of the pelvis, is a ventral ramus from L1, with its very own name, the *iliohypogastric nerve.*

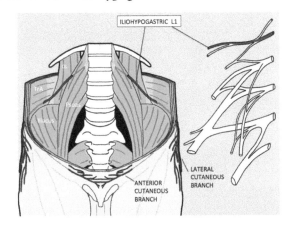

A classic patient will arrive with "lateral shift" which makes their torso look as though it has been separated from their lower body, then reapplied, but sideways by an inch or two. They will likely be in quite a lot of pain also, and likely not able to perform any range of movement testing. If you examine the top edge of the lateral pelvis in supine, you will usually find a very, very sore spot on one side, often the side toward which they are shifted but sometimes on both sides.

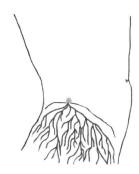

INDICATION: LATERAL SHIFT OF TRUNK WITH SHARP BACK PAIN OF SUDDEN
DURATION, ACCOMPANIED BY TENDER POINT ON TOP OF LATERAL ILIUM;
DULL BACK DISCOMFORT OF ANY DURATION WITH RESTRICTED HIP DROP

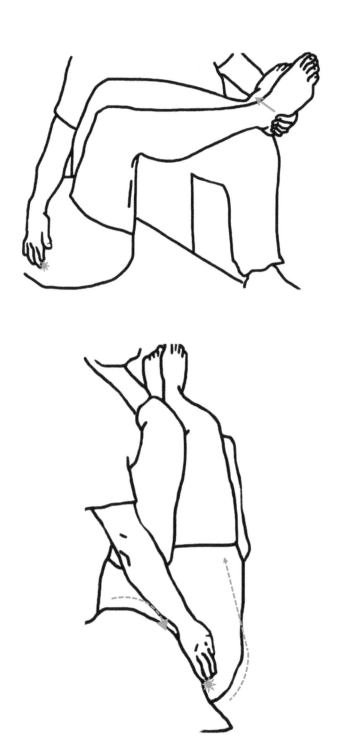

TREATMENT: POSITIONAL RELAXATION APPROACH
COMBINED WITH SKIN STRETCH

1. Ask patient to lie supine.

2. Test for tender point on top of bony pelvis, exactly lateral. If this nerve is entrapped, there will be a very sharp tender spot found there.

3. Stand on the *un*affected side of your patient.

4. Help patient to flex up both legs. Put your foot up on the table.

5. Rest patient's legs on top of your knee. Patient's legs should be at about 90 degrees of flexion at hip and knee.

6. Cross the foot on the affected side *under* foot on side closest to you, the unaffected side, if necessary.

7. Reach across, locate sore spot, monitor with one hand. With other hand, pull patients feet toward you, away from tender side. Be sure the thighs remain vertical.

8. The patient's thigh on affected side will go into slight external rotation. The tenderness should decrease somewhat.

9. Support the position with your knee. Move your hand until it wraps around the bottom of the patient's foot. Grasp the skin over the bottom end of their fibula (lateral malleolus), firmly, and then pull it caudally.

10. You should be able to feel the tender point, way up at the waist, move slightly.

11. Spot will suddenly soften and be less tender.

12. Hold for at least 2 minutes.

13. Slowly let go. Restore patient's body to a neutral position. Ask patient to stand and move. They should be able to move easier, not have to hold their trunk rigidly or off to one side. They might even be able to perform range of motion testing.

14. They may still need to be taught to actively slide their ribcage over to the side it could not go before.

TROCHANTERIC RETE

The area over the trochanter is a convergence zone for superior cluneal nerves, small cutaneous branches of iliohypogastric nerve, inferior cluneal nerves, and lateral cutaneous nerve of the thigh. As with any bony prominence, the nest of neural and vascular structure over it is called a rete. Do not forget to treat the rete. At least, consider it in your clinical reasoning.

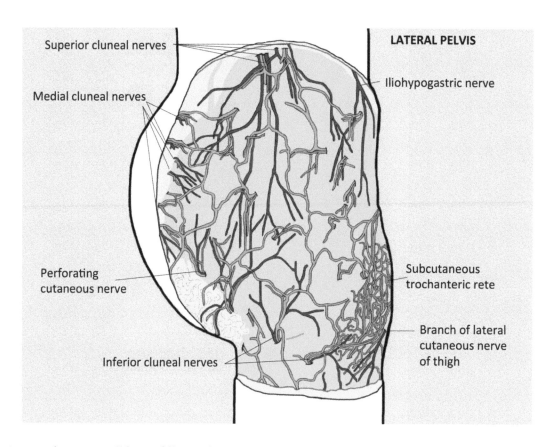

A typical patient will be middle age, have pain there, either sharp or dull, usually longstanding. It will either bother them to lie on that side, or it may feel best when laid on. In either case, the patient has usually slept mainly on one side all their life, or crossed one leg habitually but not the other. They may have been diagnosed with bursitis but never developed any swelling or redness. They may have tried injections which did not work.

In any case, here are a few treatment suggestions that seem to work fairly well for annoying pain in this area.

INDICATION: PAIN OVER OR BEHIND TROCHANTER

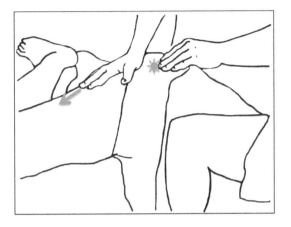

TREATMENT: SKIN STRETCH APPROACH

1. Patient is in comfortable sidelying.
2. Knee may be supported on a pillow, if necessary.
3. Locate tender point.
4. Stretch skin away from it, in any direction until you find the direction that works best.
5. When tenderness disappears, hold for a few minutes.
6. Move to next spot. Be patient. There may be many sore spots.

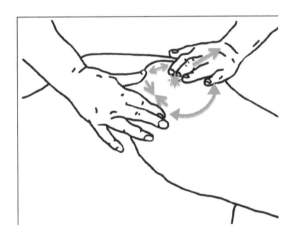

TREATMENT VARIATION: SKIN GATHERING (BALLOON APPROACH)

1. Same set-up.
2. Locate sore spot
3. Use other hand to bunch up skin while dragging tender point away with the other.

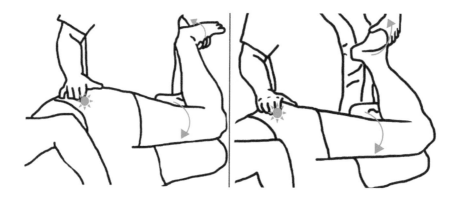

TREATMENT VARIATION: POSITIONAL RELAXATION APPROACH
COMBINED WITH 'TWIZZLE' APPROACH THROUGH FOOT

1. Patient is in comfortable sidelying, their back at edge of table, knees together and flexed. Hips may be slightly flexed.

2. Stand behind patient. Locate sore spot with one hand.

3. With other hand, grasp foot comfortably.

4. Lift the foot up into the air, leaving knee down. Thigh will go into internal rotation.

5. Take the foot into either abduction eversion, or adduction inversion, which ever way works best.

6. As soon as tenderness feels gone, hold the position for a couple minutes.

ANTERIOR PELVIS AND ANTERIOR HIP

Several nerves innervate the skin organ at the top of the thigh. The inguinal ligament poses an obstacle to all of them. As a group, they may be considered the cutaneous "inguinal nerves." They are *lateral cutaneous nerve of the thigh* (L2), *genitofemoral* (L3), *femoral* (L3-4) and *ilioinguinal* (L2) nerves.

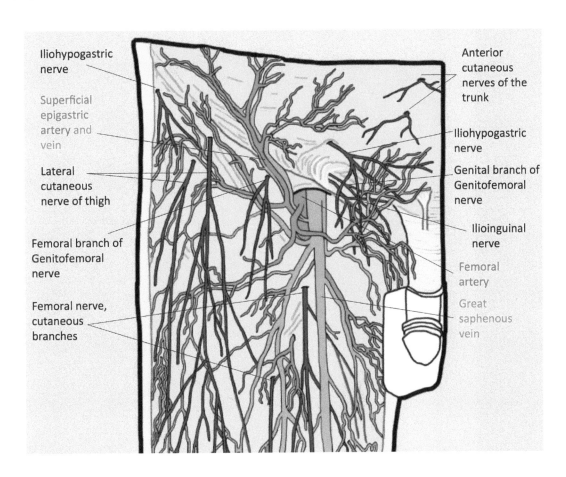

The "inguinal ligament" is not really a ligament at all: It is simply a fold in the abdominal wall; internal oblique folds diagonally to become external oblique during embryological formation. In any case, there is very little space beneath it for all these nerves and a huge femoral artery and vein to pass.

The nerves that must contend with this situation descend in front of the body wall behind abdominal contents, along psoas muscle inside the pelvis.

The best position for treating them seems to be supine with legs comfortably flexed up over a stable bolster. This brings the area into more of a quadruped position, which slackens, shortens and widens the neural container, giving the lumbosacral plexus more room to breathe.

A typical presentation will be someone who feels pain at the anterior hip, or groin, secondary to some sort of injury perhaps, which may have been decades earlier. Full hip flexion is uncomfortable for them. Often they cannot full extend the hip either. They tend to not like the way stair climbing makes their hip feel.

Treating inguinal nerves from lateral to medial seems to be the most respectful way to go about treating inguinal nerves.

LATERAL CUTANEOUS NERVE OF THE THIGH

Entrapment of this nerve has its own name – *meralgia paresthetica*. Symptoms will be tenderness or sensory symptoms down the outside aspect of the thigh.

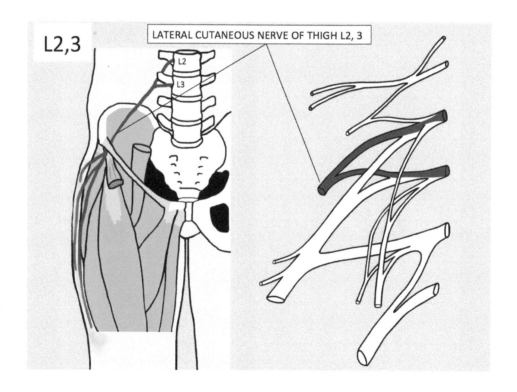

INDICATION: PAIN OR PARESTHESIA ON THE OUTSIDE OF THE
THIGH, SOMETIMES RESTRICTED HIP FLEXION OR ROTATION

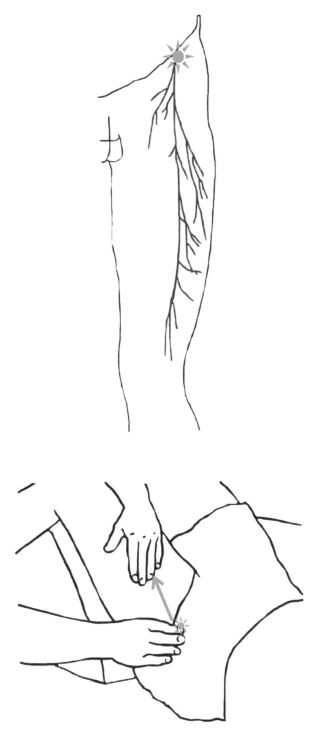

TREATMENT: POSITIONAL RELAXATION APPROACH
COMBINED WITH SKIN STRETCH

1. Patient is supine with legs relaxed over a bolster, hips in about 45 degrees of flexion.

2. Locate grommet hole where lateral cutaneous nerve of thigh emerges, medial and inferior to anterior superior iliac spine. Sometimes it will feel tender. Usually it will feel like a hard nodule. Monitor with one hand.

3. Place other hand on skin of thigh, just distal to your monitoring hand. Wait for hand to stick to skin. Gently pull skin layer distal.

4. After softening occurs, hold for about 2 minutes.

5. Let go slowly.

6. Ask patient to stand up, move around, and recheck range of motion

GENITOFEMORAL NERVE AND FEMORAL NERVE

Genitofemoral nerve has two main sections. The genital portion stays buried within the body, curving around almost to midline, where it emerges to cutaneously innervate skin on the side of the scrotum and is responsible for cremaster reflex. In females it innervates a portion of external labia.

The femoral portion innervates the large femoral artery, and a small patch of skin at the top of the thigh.

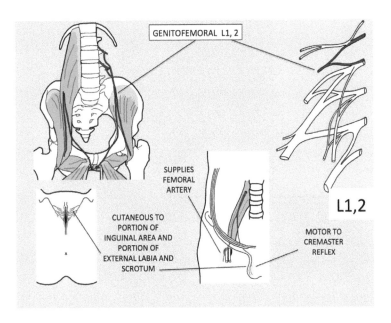

Femoral nerve is massive and massively branched; it supplies all the muscles of the front of the thigh and cutaneous branches supply all the skin on the front of the thigh, and the medial side of the lower leg, all the way down to the big toe through its saphenous branch.

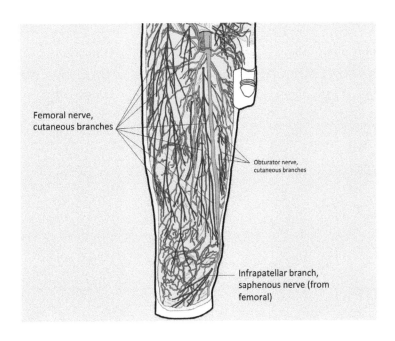

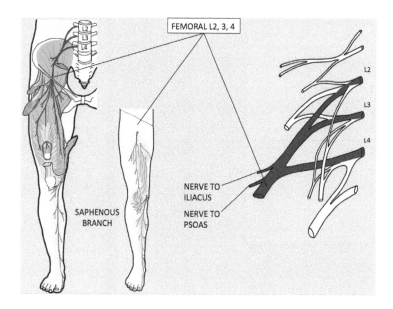

The emergence points for both femoral nerve and femoral portion of genitofemoral nerve, are close together and may be treated as one. The set-up is the same as it was for lateral cutaneous nerve of the thigh previously described. The nodules or tender spots will be found about midway between ASIS and lateral pubic tubercle, along or just below inguinal ligament.

INDICATION: PAIN OR PARESTHESIA AT FRONT OF HIP AND/OR
THIGH, SOMETIMES RESTRICTED HIP FLEXION OR ROTATION

TREATMENT: POSITIONAL RELAXATION APPROACH
COMBINED WITH SKIN STRETCH

1. Patient is supine with legs relaxed over a bolster, hips in about 45 degrees of flexion.
2. Locate area of tenderness or hardness, about halfway between ASIS and lateral pubic tubercle at inguinal crease or just below it. Monitor with one hand.
3. Place other hand on skin of thigh just distal to your monitoring hand. Wait for hand to stick to skin. Gently pull skin layer distal.
4. After softening occurs, hold for about 2 minutes.
5. Let go slowly.
6. Ask patient to stand up, move around, and recheck range of motion

ILIOINGUINAL NERVE

This nerve is the most medial of this group. As a ventral ramus from L1 and 2, it travels around the body, within the body wall, *inside* the inguinal ligament, until it emerges nearly at midline. It cutaneously innervates the skin organ over the adductor tendon and the upper medial side of the thigh. I am fairly sure that entrapment of this nerve is implicated in most so-called "groin injuries."

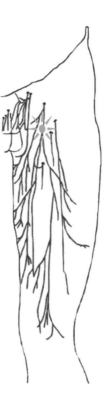

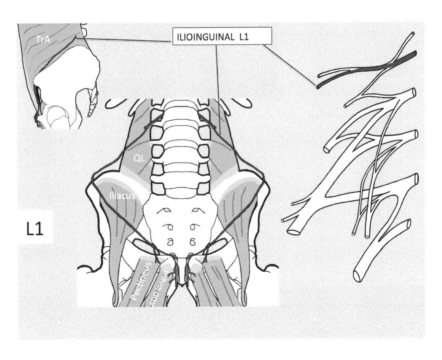

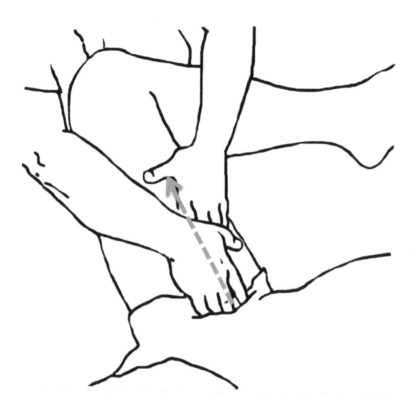

TREATMENT: POSITIONAL RELAXATION APPROACH
COMBINED WITH SKIN STRETCH

1. Patient is supine with legs relaxed over a bolster, hips in about 45 degrees of flexion.

2. Bring the affected leg up into flexion and abduction; allow lateral border of foot to rest comfortably and securely on top of the bolster. Place your body so that the patient's knee can rest against it to create a bit of slack for the nerve. This allows the adductor tendon to become prominent.

3. Explain to the patient that you want to travel up the tendon to where it joins the body, to find a sore spot there. A sore spot there will be where the nerve becomes cutaneous. It will usually be very tender. Monitor it with one hand.

4. Place other hand on skin of thigh just distal to your monitoring hand, on the skin overlying the tendon. Wait for hand to stick to skin. Gently pull skin layer distal. The tenderness will usually disappear, abruptly.

5. After tenderness disappears, be still and hold for about 2 minutes.

6. Let go slowly.

7. Ask patient to stand up, move around, and recheck range of motion

ILIOHYPOGASTRIC NERVE, anterior branch, and SUBCOSTAL NERVE (T12), both travel around the body wall to the front as well. They do not have to contend with the inguinal ligament however. They emerge close to midline above the pubic bone.

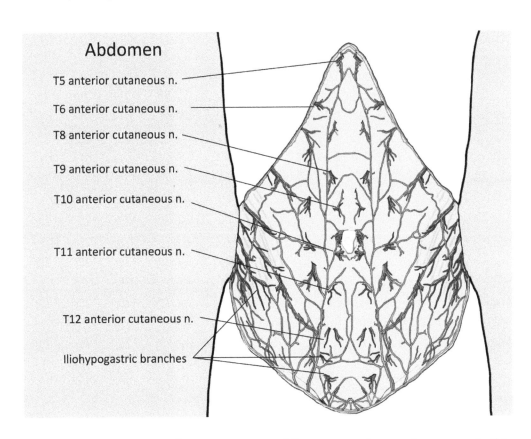

Entrapment of these nerves may be a consequence of Cesarean section or other surgery in this area. Do what you can think of to treat non-medical pain associated with these nerves in the low abdominal area. I teach people to stretch their own skin in this region as it is usually easy for them to reach; both hands, let skin attach to skin, pull skin up toward head, breathe slowly and move skin only on exhale, hold for a few minutes, take up any slack that presents itself. Done carefully, one can feel one's skin stretch down as far as the knees.

POSTERIOR AND MEDIAL SIDE OF THIGH AND KNEE

Two main cutaneous nerves supply the skin organ of the posterior and medial sides of the thigh, *posterior cutaneous nerve of the thigh*, and *obturator*.

POSTERIOR CUTANEOUS NERVE OF THE THIGH

This nerve is massive and massively branched. Some of its branches are independently named; we will address them separately later.

The main part going down the back of the leg has multiple grommet holes and descends beyond the knee crease to the lower leg. Pain felt at the back of the thigh is often blamed on the sciatic nerve; however, this *cutaneous* nerve may be associated with pain at back of thigh also. It is easy to access with simple skin stretch which can ease a lot of discomfort, stiffness, pain, and restricted straight leg raise felt there.

A typical patient may have experienced pain at the back of their thigh for years. They usually have no back pain or difficulties moving their spine. They may feel increased discomfort if you test their straight leg raise, and it may be limited on the affected side, sometimes both sides.

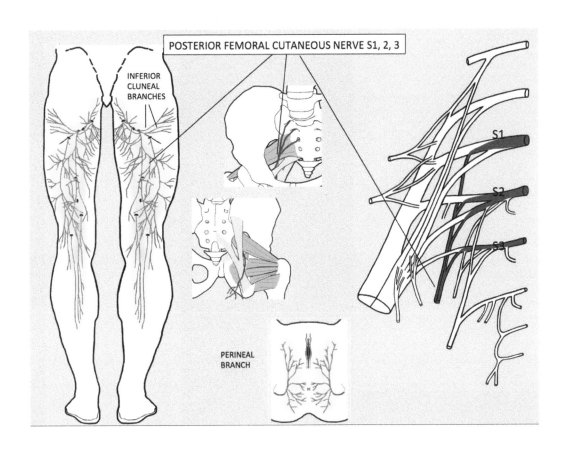

POSTERIOR FEMORAL CUTANEOUS NERVE S1, 2, 3

INFERIOR CLUNEAL BRANCHES

PERINEAL BRANCH

S1

S2

S3

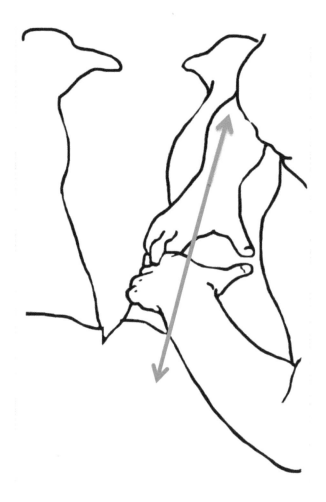

TREATMENT: SKIN STRETCH APPROACH

1. Patient is prone. Be sure that feet and toes are resting on the bed.

2. Spread elbows apart, place forearms and hands on skin of posterior leg. Let hands and arms stick to skin. Elbows should point directly away from each other.

3. Slowly pull elbows apart, drawing skin longitudinally.

4. Hold for about 2 minutes, let go slowly. Adapt to any changes you may feel within the thigh.

5. Ask patient to stand up and move about, check amount and quality of range, whether pain has decreased.

OBTURATOR NERVE

The obturator nerve innervates several structures inside the pelvis, including the hip joint and some small hip muscles. It emerges through the obturator foramen down the medial side of the thigh. About a third of people have an accessory branch which descends in front of the superior ramus of the pelvis. If it is there you will not know, but by treating the inguinal nerves carefully, you will include this branch with that group. Outside the pelvis, obturator nerve provides motor innervation to adductor muscles. It supplies a fairly large area of skin on medial thigh between pelvis and knee.

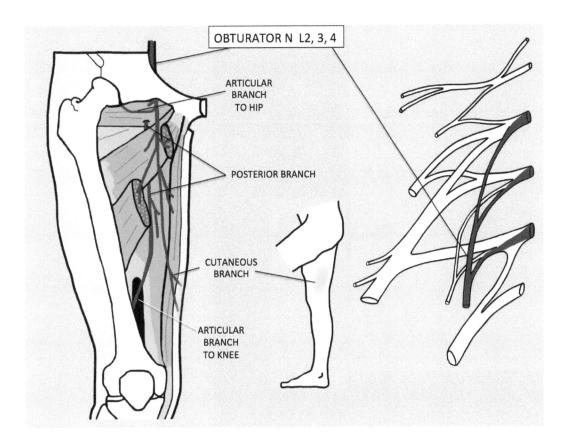

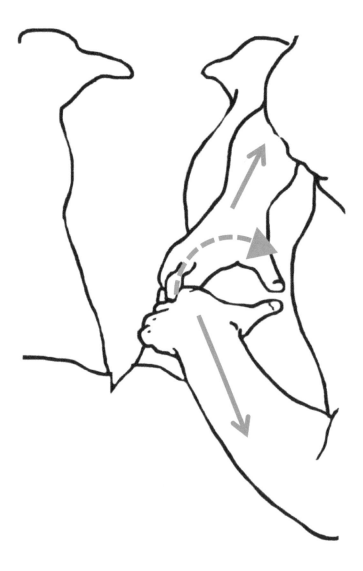

TREATMENT: SKIN STRETCH APPROACH

1. Patient is prone. Be sure that feet and toes are resting on the bed.
2. Spread elbows apart, place forearms on skin of posterior leg. Let hands and arms stick to skin. Elbows should point directly away from each other.
3. Place both hands around medial side of leg, above knee. Let hands and arms stick to skin.
4. Slowly pull elbows apart, drawing skin longitudinally, and at the same time, lift the skin above knee into medial rotation around the leg.
5. Hold for about 2 minutes, let go slowly.
6. Ask patient to stand up and move about, check amount and quality of range, whether pain has decreased.

PELVIC FLOOR

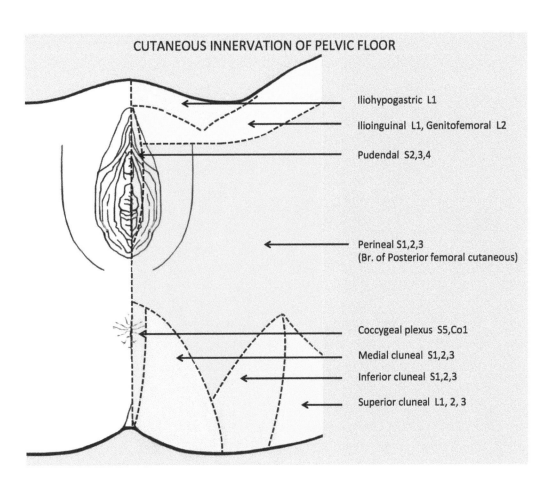

CUTANEOUS INNERVATION OF PELVIC FLOOR

Iliohypogastric L1

Ilioinguinal L1, Genitofemoral L2

Pudendal S2,3,4

Perineal S1,2,3
(Br. of Posterior femoral cutaneous)

Coccygeal plexus S5,Co1

Medial cluneal S1,2,3

Inferior cluneal S1,2,3

Superior cluneal L1, 2, 3

All the cutaneous nerves of the lower body converge to supply the skin organ of the bottom of the trunk, the pelvic floor.

Cutaneous supply to the skin organ of the pelvic floor is by the easily accessible **perineal nerve,** a branch of the posterior cutaneous nerve of the thigh. For treatment purposes we include the **coccygeal plexus** in with the perineal nerve. We will start at the posterior pelvic floor with **inferior cluneal nerves,** also branches of the posterior cutaneous nerve of the thigh, and work our way forward.

INFERIOR CLUNEAL NERVES:

These branches of the large posterior cutaneous nerve of the thigh sweep upward to supply the skin organ at the bottom of the buttocks.

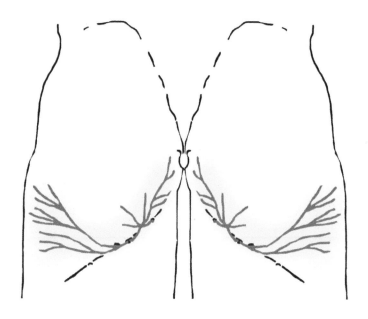

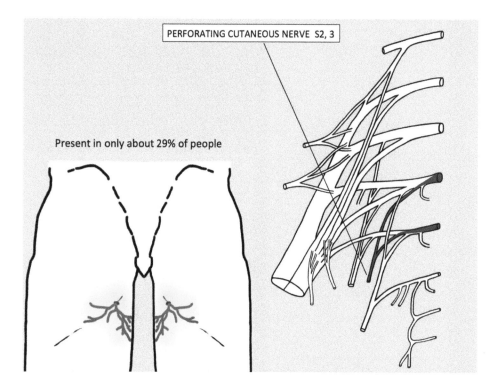

Perforating cutaneous nerve is an accessory nerve, estimated to be present in just under a third of the population.

A typical patient will have a job sitting, maybe twisting to one side all the time. They will complain of longstanding pain in one buttock only, which may extend to pelvic floor. You will be able to locate tenderness at the ischial tuberosity or just medial to it. Sitting aggravates the pain.

INDICATION: PAIN FELT AT ISCHIAL TUBEROSITY WHILE SITTING

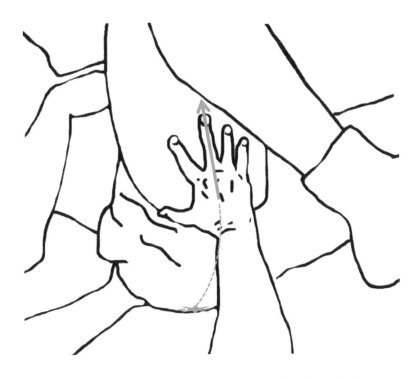

TREATMENT: POSITIONAL RELAXATION APPROACH
COMBINED WITH SKIN STRETCH

1. Patient is supine. Legs are comfortably supported over a bolster.

2. Flex leg on the side to be treated, up into about 90 degrees hip flexion. Bring the patient's foot up to rest securely up on the top of the bolster.

3. Slide one hand behind the buttock, and locate the ischial tuberosity. Find the tender point near there, just medial usually.

4. Place other hand against skin behind thigh, heel of hand near the ischial tuberosity, fingers pointing toward patient's knee.

5. Wait until skin and hand stick together. Use a piece of dycem, or some other sticky material, if necessary. Slowly pull skin layer up toward knee. This will take some time – do not be in a hurry. Sore spot will soften, tenderness will decrease.

6. Once tenderness is gone, wait 2 minutes, and then slowly let go.

7. Ask patient to get up, check for changes in quality of movement, ability to sit comfortably.

PERINEAL NERVE

The **perineal nerve**, a branch of the posterior femoral cutaneous nerve of thigh, sweeps medially into the skin of the pelvic floor. Entrapment of this nerve can be responsible for a great deal of pelvic floor pain, in my opinion. It may be treated along with the coccygeal plexus.

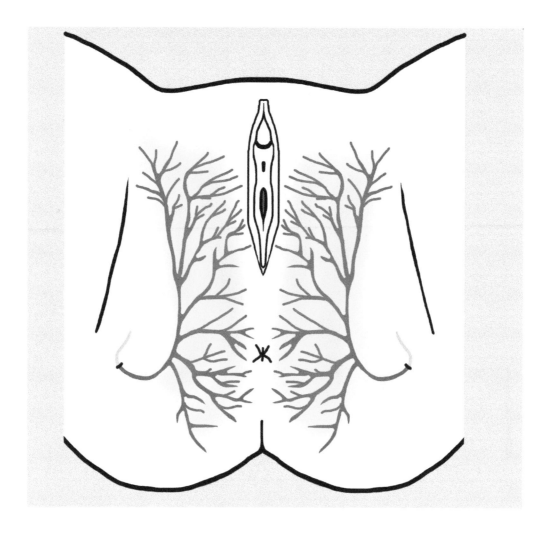

COCCYGEAL PLEXUS

The **Coccygeal plexus** is a small nest of nerves that supplies the skin over the end of the tailbone and around the outside of the anus. A patient may sit at work, but not feel pain except at night located at the end of the tailbone and anus, when they lying in bed, not sitting.

After I treat patients with this problem, I usually give them a piece of dycem to take home, and teach them how to treat themselves.

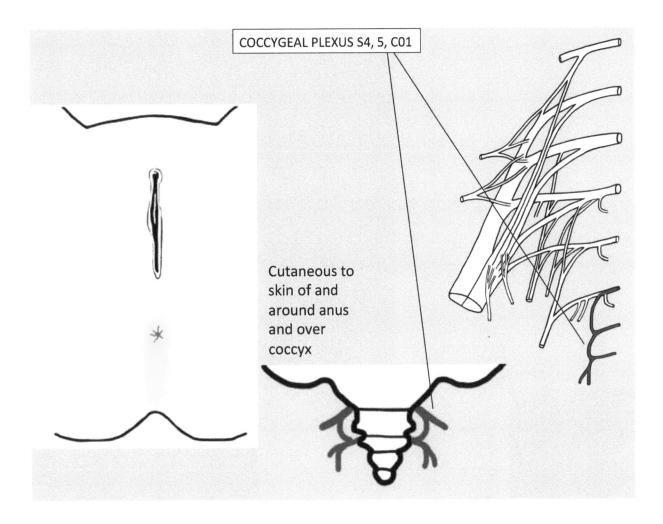

COCCYGEAL PLEXUS S4, 5, C01

Cutaneous to skin of and around anus and over coccyx

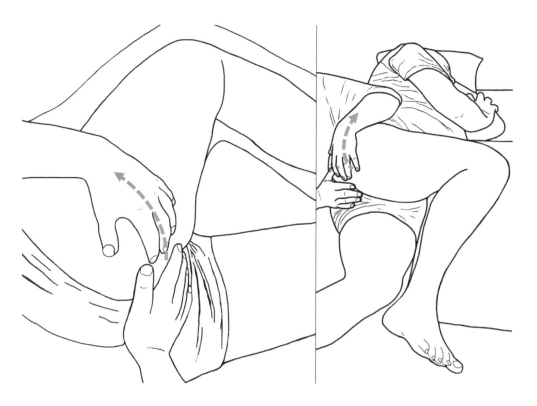

TREATMENT: SKIN STRETCH APPROACH

1. Establish good treatment boundaries by explaining exactly what you want to do, why, where your hands will be, beforehand. Ask for permission before proceeding.

2. Patient may wear thin underwear. Patient lies on one side, top leg comfortably resting on a pillow or bolster.

3. Entire pelvic floor may feel excruciatingly tender, so be careful. Therapist places one hand gently on pelvic floor.

4. If you are addressing the perineal nerve, leaving your hand in contact will activate warm thermoreceptors and will not be experienced as nociceptive.

5. If you are addressing anal pain or tailbone pain, find a tender point at the tip of tailbone, but do not hurt it.

6. With other hand, therapist gently/slowly pulls skin away from pelvic floor/anus, until a slight tug indicates "far enough". Tenderness will disappear, usually quite rapidly. Hold for 2 minutes or as long as necessary.

7. Take hands away gently. Ask patient to rise and move around, sit, check for change in discomfort in sitting.

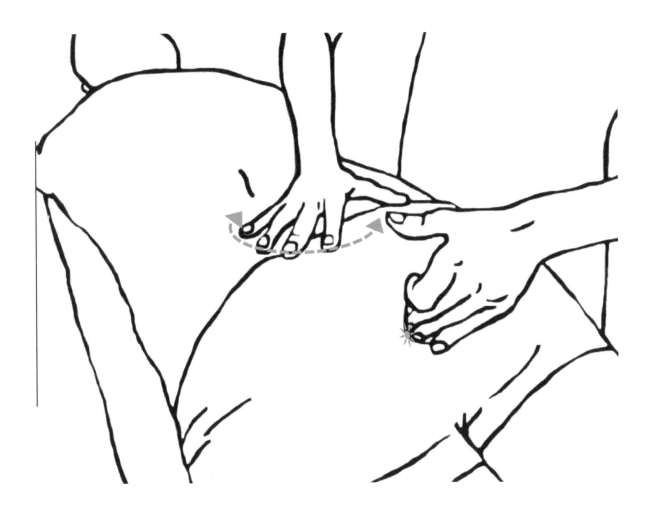

1. Patient is prone. Bring legs into slight abduction and internal rotation to access the coccyx. Light clothing may be worn.

2. With one hand locate the tip of the coccyx.

3. Place the other hand, flat, directly on the skin over the sacrum. Pressure may be used. Pressure over the sacrum feels good, and will help relax the structures below.

4. You may feel the tip of the coccyx extend a bit more from its usual tucked position.

5. To each side of the tip of coccyx palpate for tenderness. One side will usually be more tender than the other. Choose the side that is the most tender.

6. Twist the skin over the sacrum slowly, either clockwise or counterclockwise. Work with the patient to determine which way feels best to them. Also palpate for softening; usually the direction that provides the most relief of tenderness also results in the most softening.

7. Once tenderness has decreased by a lot, hold the torque and pressure for at least two minutes.

8. Repeat other side if necessary.

PUDENDAL NERVE

The pelvic floor is comprised of *two* structural floors; the main nerve serving both is the **pudendal nerve** of the sacral plexus. It is motor to all the supportive musculature there, which remains in tonic contraction to contain all the pelvic viscera, and to all the muscle and vasculature responsible for continence, elimination, and all the sensory input and motor output of sexual arousal and climax, including all the hydraulics. The only cutaneous portion of the pudendal nerve is to skin over dorsal clitoris and dorsal penis.

Pudendal nerve is enclosed within a fibro osseous tunnel known as Alcock's Canal.

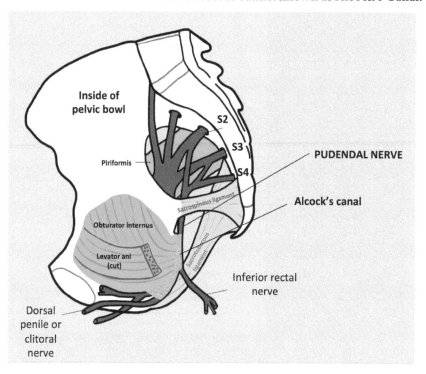

Childbirth poses a risk to the pudendal nerve. Sexual assault can injure it. Narrow seats on bicycles, or a hard fall onto the pelvis, can result in a tunnel syndrome.

Non-medical pelvic floor pain with or without incontinence is common. An entire branch of physiotherapy has developed to deal with it. If your patient presents with more than just a simple pain problem, you may need to refer to a pelvic health PT.

For women, entrapment of pudendal nerve is implicated if there is pain during sexual intercourse. For men, entrapment of the pudendal nerve is implicated if they complain of feeling a sensation like a spiked golf ball inside the rectum; they may have received antibiotic treatment for "prostatitis," which did not help the discomfort.

The nerve is deep inside the pelvis. The only contact for those of us not certified to do internal work is to approach the nerve externally; indirect contact through other tissue is possible, medial to ischial tuberosity and over the inferior ramus. Treatment can be done in sidelying, which feels less invasive. Occasionally it may be better to treat in supine; the sacrum will be more compressed, which possibly shortens and slackens the neural container for the sacral plexus slightly.

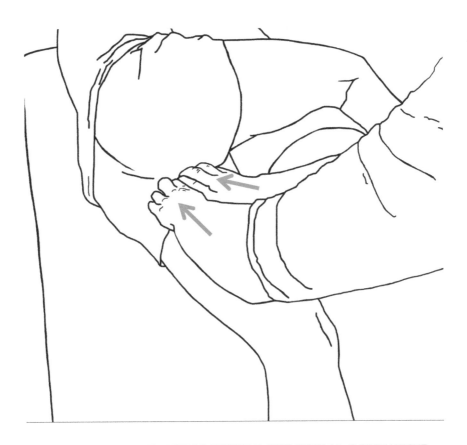

TREATMENT: DIRECT PRESSURE ON NEURAL CONTAINER

1. Establish good treatment boundaries beforehand. Point out structures you intend to touch on a skeletal model, if possible.

2. Patient may wear thin underwear. Patient lies on one side, top leg over a pillow.

3. Therapist places both hands, or just one, on the ischial tuberosity of the lower limb.

4. Slowly insert straight fingers into soft tissue of pelvic floor just medial to ischial tuberosity and over the inferior ramus. Hold for many minutes. Go slowly through several stages. Eventually pelvic floor will soften. When it feels as though no more softening is likely to occur, withdraw hand slowly.

5. Ask patient to rise and move around, sit, check for change in discomfort in sitting.

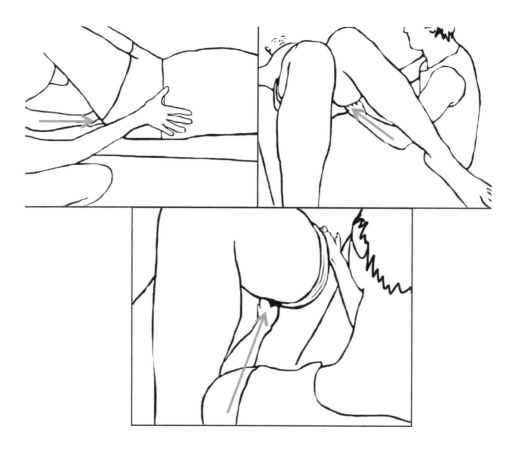

1. Establish good treatment boundaries beforehand. Patient may wear thin underwear. Patient is supine, hips flexed about 60 degrees, knees supported against each other, feet apart, legs relaxed. Ask patient to breathe somewhat slower and deeper than usual.

2. One hand rests against side of pelvis to reassure and to monitor breathing.

3. With the other hand locate ischial tuberosity. Move just medial to it. Ensure wrist is straight and arm is lined up parallel to patient's body

4. Slowly insert straight fingers into soft tissue of pelvic floor just medial to ischial tuberosity and over inferior ramus. Hold for many minutes. Go slowly through several stages. Eventually pelvic floor will soften. Withdraw hand slowly.

5. Ask patient to rise and move around, sit, check for change in discomfort in sitting.

KNEE AND LOWER LEG

ANTERIOR KNEE AND MEDIAL LEG

Femoral Cutaneous Nerves

Nerves of anterior knee are mainly **cutaneous branches of femoral nerve.**

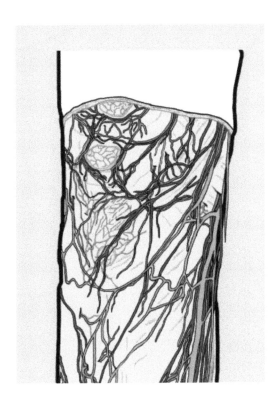

Rete in front of the patella.

One can treat the rete over the patella and all the cutaneous nerves as a group, simply by pulling skin there, slowly and gently, in any number of different ways, twisting it gently, etc.

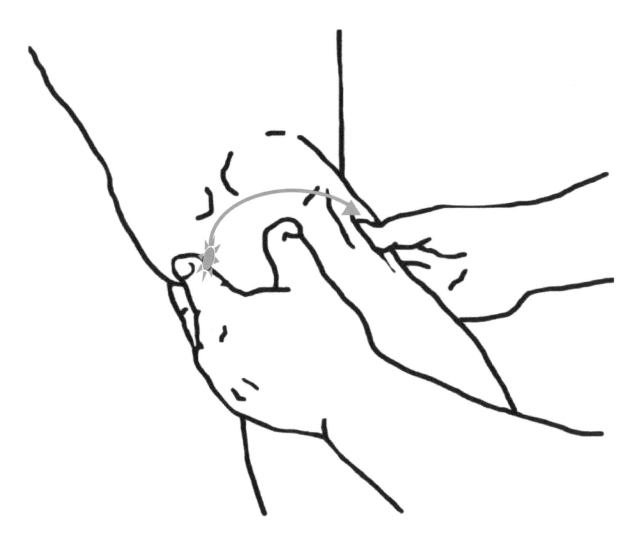

TREATMENT: SKIN STRETCH APPROACH

1. Patient is supine. Knee is extended.

2. With one hand, locate tender point anywhere on knee. In the image we can see the tender point is on the medial side of the knee, but it could be anywhere. Find it, then monitor only.

3. With other hand, draw skin over front of knee toward whatever direction results in decreased tenderness, using patella as a fulcrum. Proceed slowly.

4. After softening and maximum decreased tenderness is achieved, hold at least 2 minutes. Slowly let go. Tenderness should remain gone.

5. Ask patient to stand and reevaluate movement, range, discomfort level.

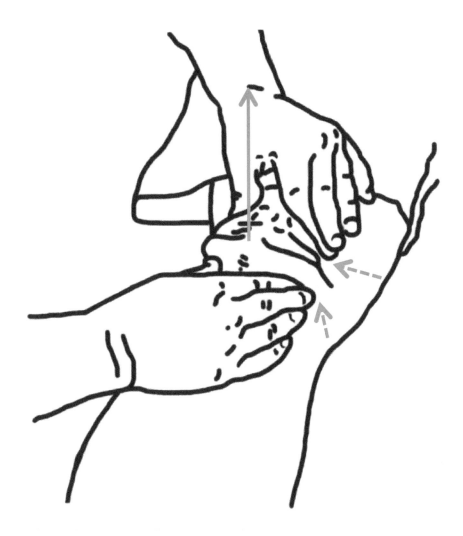

1. Patient is supine. Knee is extended.

2. Place one hand above, and the other below, the patella.

3. Slowly, with a great deal of attention to any physiological changes you can sense through your hands, draw skin into a wrinkled mass over the patella. Do not press down, instead lift, as though you were trying to lift the patella itself from all sides. Proceed slowly. Try to create several deep wrinkles.

4. This will usually feel very pleasant to the patient. After softening and maximum decreased tenderness is achieved, hold at least 2 minutes. Slowly let go. Tenderness should remain gone.

5. Ask patient to stand and reevaluate movement, range, discomfort level.

One long branch of the femoral nerve, the saphenous nerve, remains buried in a canal inside the thigh until it reaches the medial knee. There, it gives off a cutaneous *infrapatellar branch*, and a *cutaneous posterior branch,* both of which deserve specific treatment. The rest of the saphenous nerve supplies the skin organ for the medial leg and medial side of foot.

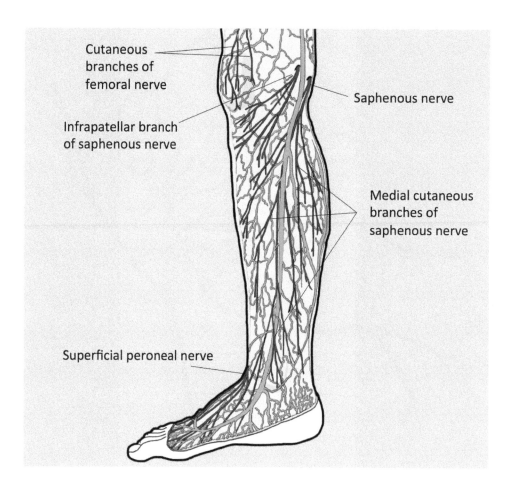

Infrapatellar Branch of Saphenous Nerve:

This branch emerges at the medial knee and swoops laterally to innervate the skin below the knee. A typical case will be someone with medial knee pain of any duration and a feeling that they cannot fully extend or straighten the knee. A limp is almost inevitable. Stair climbing will be painful. The knee will not have that last few degrees of passive locking stability, so gait will be slowed.

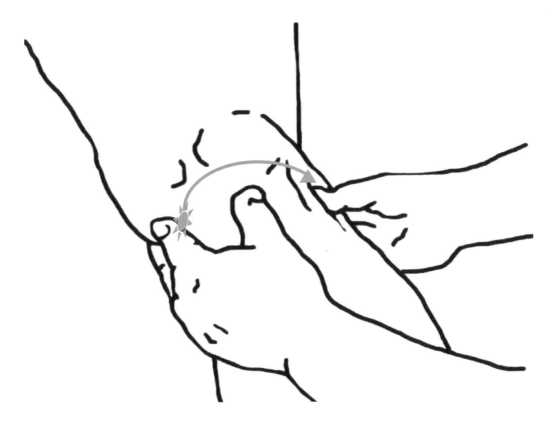

TREATMENT: SKIN STRETCH APPROACH

Treatment is targeted to wherever the nerve surfaces, usually at the medial joint line or just above. One may have to treat with skin pull in several other directions, as the nerve is multiply branched and more than just the main grommet hole may be involved. See previous treatment images.

Posterior Branch of Saphenous Nerve

Treatment of the posterior branch is every bit as important to regaining knee function as treatment of the infrapatellar branch.

INDICATION: MEDIAL KNEE PAIN OF ANY DURATION THAT
INTERFERES WITH KNEE MOVEMENT AND USE

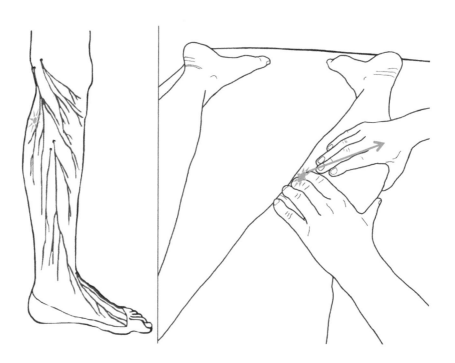

TREATMENT: SKIN STRETCH APPROACH

1. Patient is prone. Make sure toes are resting on and supported by the bed.
2. Locate tender point with one finger, monitor only.
3. Place forearm of other arm against the back of the leg, as shown, below knee. Let hands and arms stick to skin.
4. Slowly draw the skin in the direction the nerve disseminates, drawing skin longitudinally away from knee crease. You may also need to lift the skin above knee into medial rotation around the leg.
5. Feel all the activity going on physiologically under your hands. There will be a lot of fasciculation happening, usually. This will feel as though it dies down, eventually.
6. Hold for about 2 more minutes, and then let go slowly.
7. Ask patient to stand up, recheck movement, quality of range.

POSTERIOR KNEE

The back and lateral side of the lower leg is supplied by several branches of the *sciatic nerve*. The three main nerves are the *tibial nerve* (which is just the sciatic nerve with a change of name as it crosses the back of the knee joint), the *peroneal nerve*, (deep and superficial) and the cutaneous *sural nerve*.

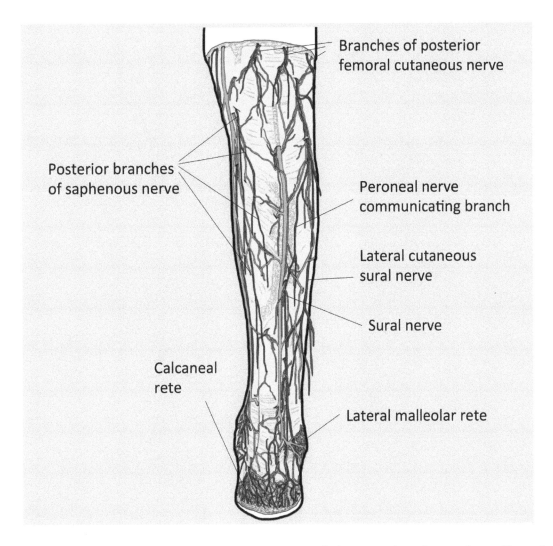

Branches of posterior femoral cutaneous nerve

Posterior branches of saphenous nerve

Peroneal nerve communicating branch

Lateral cutaneous sural nerve

Sural nerve

Calcaneal rete

Lateral malleolar rete

In the foot, the tibial nerve becomes the *plantar nerve*, with three main branches – *calcaneal branch, medial and lateral branch.* The skin organ over the lateral side of the leg and foot is supplied mainly by the sural nerve. The skin organ over the bottom of the foot is supplied by cutaneous branches of the plantar nerve.

Tibial Nerve:

As can be seen in the following image, the tibial nerve has to pierce through muscle on its way down to the foot. Not shown are the substantial vascular structures that accompany it. A branch from this nerve supplies the knee joint.

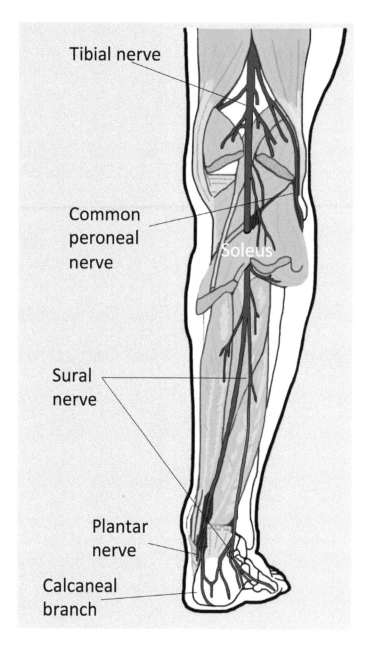

People who sit for a living may lose easy slide of this nerve through tissue over time. They may experience pain at the back of the knee, which spreads throughout the knee as a pain or ache. They may lose some knee extension or ability to lock the knee in hyperextension during walk cycle. Before somebody thinks they have to go get a total knee replacement, there is a non-surgical approach you can try.

DermoNeuroModulating | Diane Jacobs

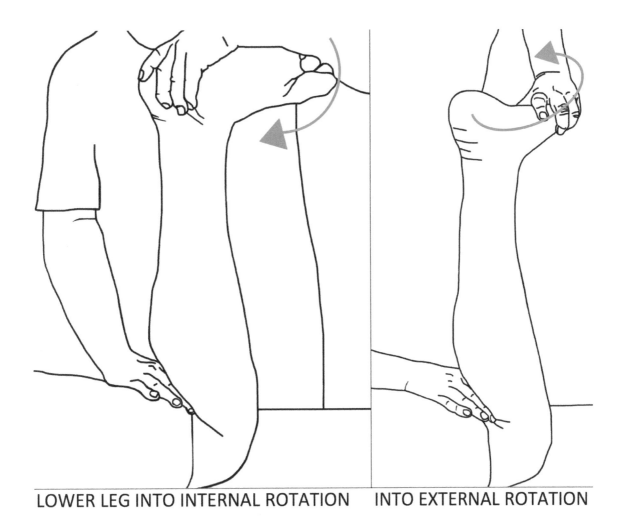

LOWER LEG INTO INTERNAL ROTATION   INTO EXTERNAL ROTATION

TREATMENT: POSITIONAL RELAXATION APPROACH,
COMBINED WITH TWIZZLE APPROACH

1. Patient is prone. Locate tender spot with one hand. Use other hand to carefully bend lower leg up to about 90 to 100 degrees or even a bit more if necessary.

2. At some indeterminable amount of flexion, the tenderness will lessen but not disappear. Maintain that amount of flexion.

3. Torque the foot to rotate the lower leg into either external or internal rotation, carefully. This should help some more.

4. Carefully add some weight through the foot to compress down through the leg, maintaining flexion and rotation. Tenderness will disappear completely. Hold for 2 minutes.

5. Decompress slowly, then slowly and securely bring the leg down onto the bed. We do not want the patient to contract at the knee during the descent.

6. Ask patient to stand up, reassess comfortable range

ANTERIOR LEG

Skin stretch approaches can be used on the front of the leg. Directional preferences I have noticed are depicted below:

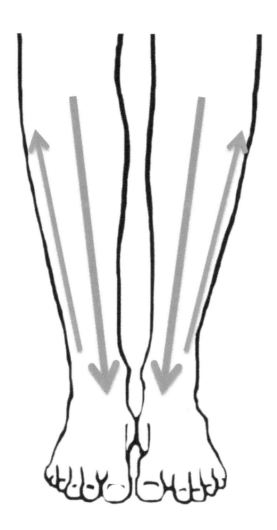

Taking skin over the front of the leg in these two directions, simultaneously, one hand moving it distally and the other hand moving it proximally, feels very good.

Peroneal Nerve:

The branches of the peroneal or fibular nerve supply all the muscles on the lateral side of the leg. Before it splits up, it winds forward and down around the head of the fibula, where it can become entrapped. Symptoms can include pain in lateral leg, ankle, or top of foot.

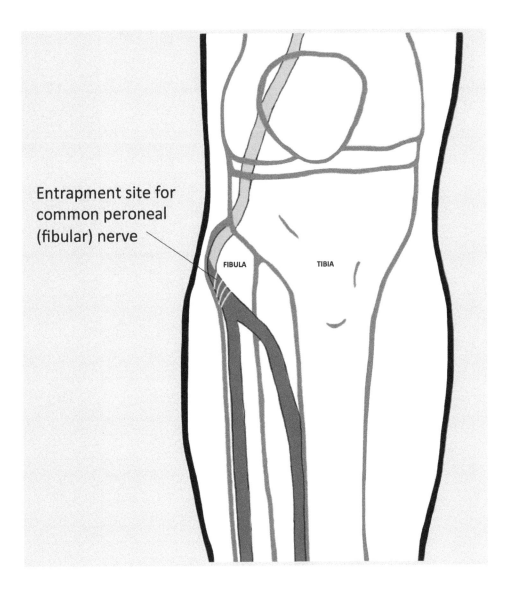

Entrapment site for common peroneal (fibular) nerve

FIBULA   TIBIA

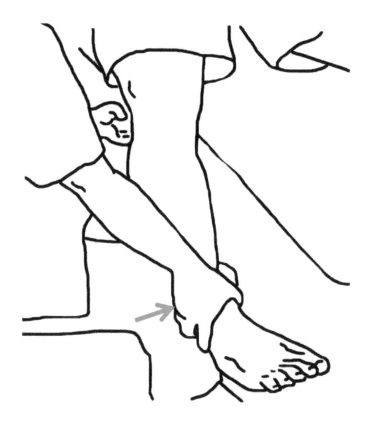

TREATMENT: POSITIONAL RELAXATION APPROACH
COMBINED WITH SKIN STRETCH

1. Patient is supine. Locate tender spot, which may be at side of leg or behind knee.

2. Bring leg down off side of bed. Hip is in extension, and about 30 degrees abduction, knee about 45 degrees flexion. Rest the patient's heel on your knee.

3. The edge of the table will act as a fulcrum for the medial side of the tibia.

4. Place other hand on skin over lateral side of ankle.

5. Slowly press ankle slightly medially. You do NOT need to use much force. You have huge mechanical advantage. The idea is to lever the tibia, and therefore the fibula, outward by a tiny bit, to affect the neural tunnel.

6. Wherever you are palpating will soften and become less tender.

7. If necessary, add some skin stretch to help tenderness decrease completely: Slide skin over the ankle into slight medial rotation. Top of tibia will be held still by edge of bed. Spot will soften and feel non-tender.

8. Hold for 2 minutes. Let go slowly. Bring leg up into neutral, on top of bed.

9. Ask patient to stand up and move around, reassess range of movement.

POSTERIOR LEG

Directional preferences I have noticed for the skin over posterior leg:

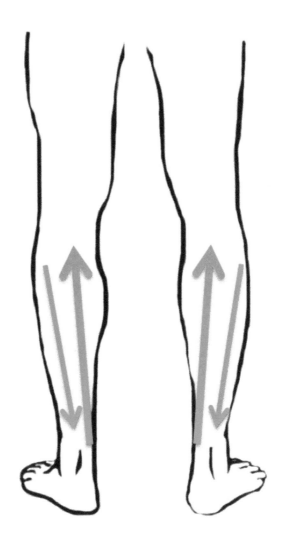

Sural Nerve:

This cutaneous nerve runs along down the back and lateral side of the leg and foot. Its branches innervate skin organ and also the Achilles tendon beneath the skin organ.

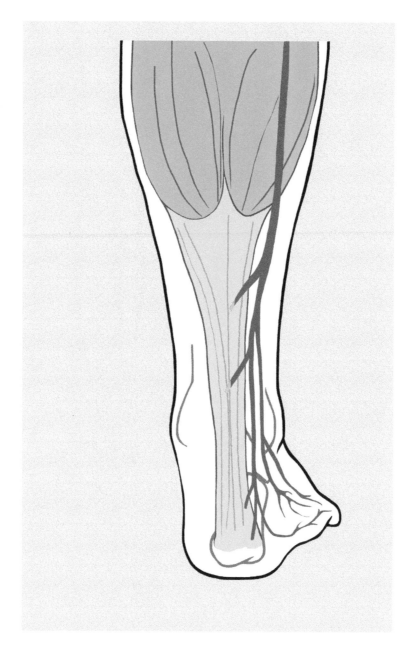

Sural nerve helps innervate the lateral side of Achilles tendon

Treatment may include skin stretch longitudinally along the course of the nerve, or ballooning around the leg to unload the nerve and its rami.

Here are a few more ideas on how to address pain over the Achilles tendon or posterior leg.

INDICATION: PAIN AT BACK OF LEG, BEHIND ANKLE

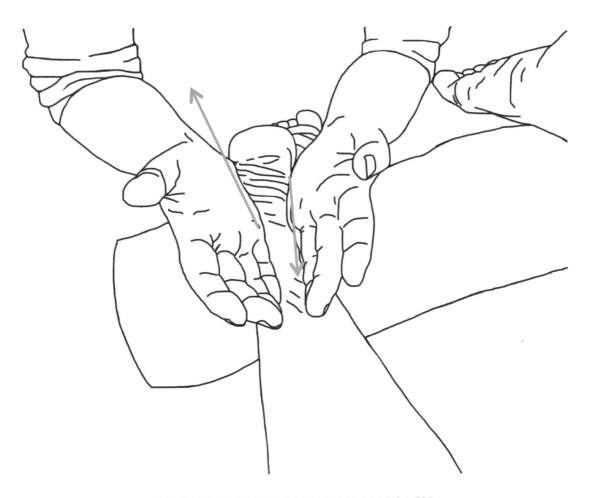

TREATMENT: SKIN STRETCH APPROACH

1. Patient is prone. Toes are resting on and supported by the bed. Ankle may be supported over a towel roll.
2. Using lateral borders of hands, gently grasp skin on both sides of Achilles tendon.
3. Wait for hands to stick to skin. Slowly pull skin layer on lateral side of tendon distally. Slowly pull skin layer on medial side of tendon, proximally.
4. Feel the physiology and fasciculation that may occur and wait for it to ebb.
5. Continue for another two minutes.
6. Bring the skin back to its resting position, then slowly and carefully remove hands.
7. Ask patient to sit up on treatment table, and move feet around in circles a few times before weight bearing.
8. Ask patient to stand, test movement and comfort level by walking on toes, performing heel drop, etc.

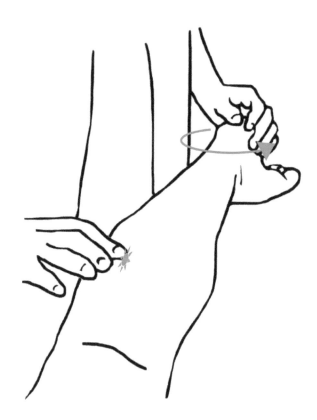

TREATMENT: POSITIONAL RELAXATION APPROACH,
COMBINED WITH SKIN STRETCH APPROACH

1. Patient is prone. Toes are resting on and supported by the bed; foot is in full plantar flexion.

2. Find tender spot on back of leg, over sural nerve or at ankle, or wherever a tender spot may be, usually near front or back of distal fibula.

3. With other hand, gently grasp skin over heel.

4. Wait for hand to stick to skin over heel. Slowly pull skin layer around heel, either clockwise or counterclockwise, whichever direction seems to result in most reduction in tenderness. It will feel very, very good to someone with chronic ankle or heel pain. A lot of pressure may feel good also.

5. Heel will move with its tightly adhered skin.

6. Twist slowly, by stages. Hold at least 2 minutes. Let go slowly

7. Ask patient to sit up on treatment table, and move feet around in circles a few times before weight bearing.

8. Ask patient to stand, test movement and comfort level by walking on toes, performing heel drop, etc.

FOOT AND ANKLE

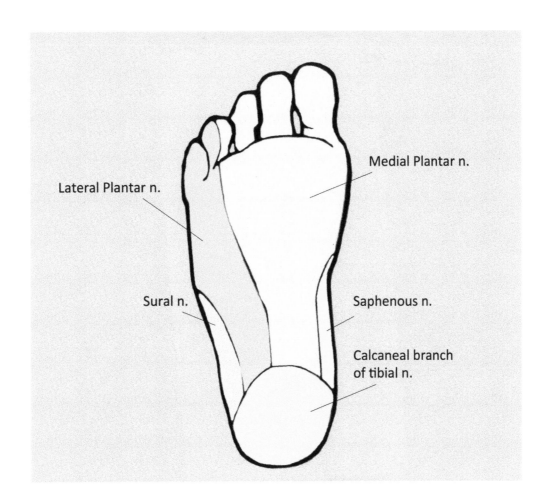

Cutaneous innervation of the sole of the foot

In the foot, the tibial nerve becomes medial and lateral plantar nerves, and calcaneal nerve.

The skin along the medial side of the foot is innervated by the long saphenous nerve, from the femoral nerve. Distal branches originating from sciatic nerve innervate the the rest of the skin of the sole of the foot including toes.

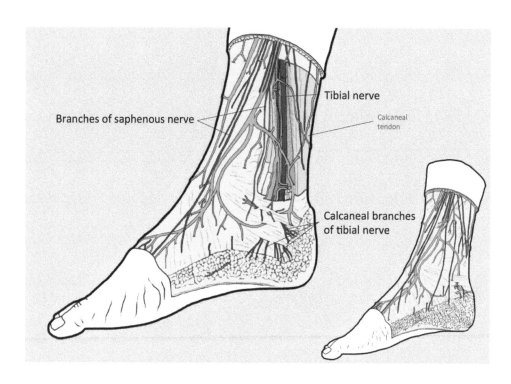

Nerves in medial side of foot and ankle.

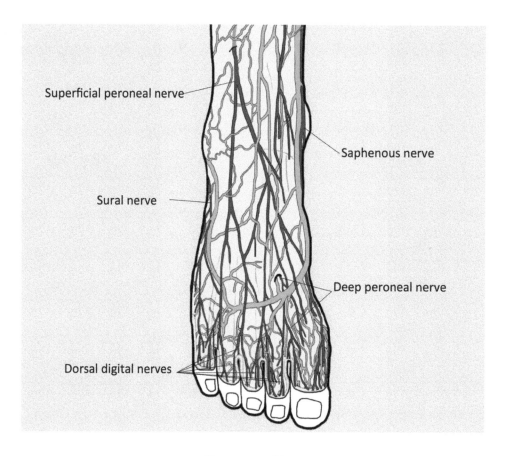

Nerves in top of foot.

The skin along the lateral border of the foot is innervated by the sural nerve, a cutaneous branch of the tibial nerve.

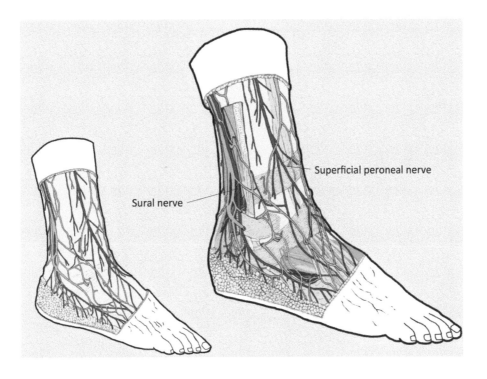

Nerves in lateral side of foot and ankle.

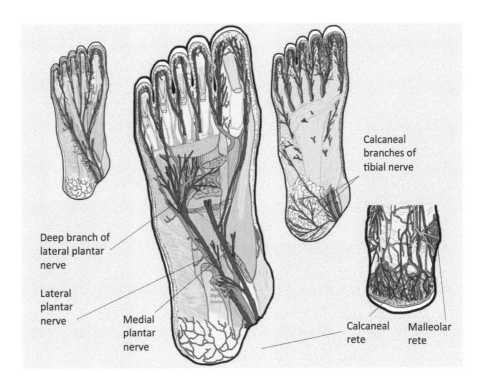

Nerves in bottom of foot and heel.

After treating feet for many years, these are the directional preferences for skin of the feet that I have noticed.

DIRECTIONAL PREFERENCES

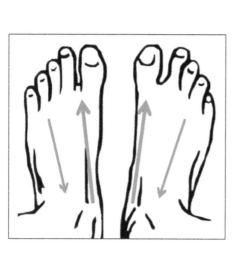
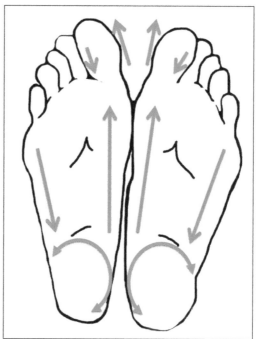

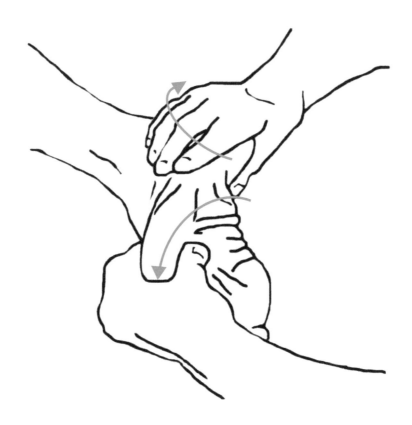

DermoNeuroModulating | Diane Jacobs

The circular arrows going both ways around the heels indicate no preference there; if heels had an opinion, it would be that they love the skin over them to be twisted in either direction.

When you look at the amount of neural content in the soles of feet in each of four main layers, you simply cannot go wrong bending feet about - the plantar nerves are going to greatly benefit by being moved.

Pain in the sole of the foot seems to be relieved best by approximating heel to toes for long enough to create deep, blanched wrinkles in the bottom of the foot. You will see the skin turn pale as the blood is driven out. The longer you can hold the foot in a wrinkled state, the better the results seem to be, even for long-standing chronic foot pain. Wringing out a wet mop by hand comes to mind as a treatment metaphor.

The classic case is someone who was told they had plantar fasciitis. When they get up in the morning the first few steps are agony, as though they were walking on little shards of glass. It gets better as they move about but they are rarely if ever pain free.

PLANTAR NERVES:

INDICATION: PAIN BOTTOM OF FOOT, MAY HAVE BEEN DIAGNOSED WITH "PLANTAR FASCIITIS"

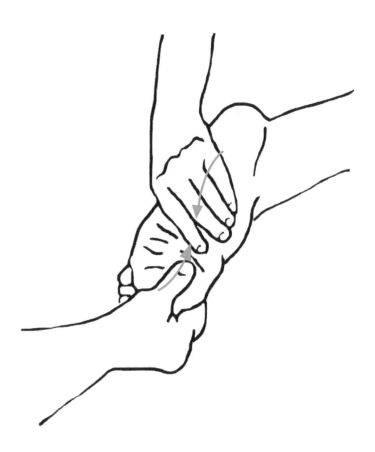

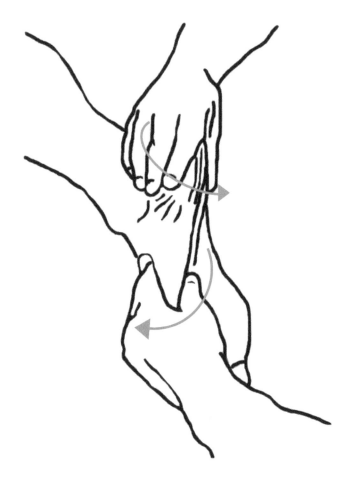

1. Patient is prone. Toes are resting on, and supported by, the table.

2. Mobilize multi-directionally.

3. Go slowly in whatever direction of ease presents itself. Hold for long periods of time. Take a good five to 7 minutes to make your way into, sustain, and then back out of, each hold.

4. Create large pale wrinkles on the bottom of the foot.

5. Increase torque force as/when system permits.

6. After 20 minutes to a half hour of this, gently and slowly let go.

7. Ask the patient to sit up, with feet over side, and move and stretch their feet and toes.

8. When they weight bear they will usually remark that there is a large decrease in foot pain. They may mention that the feet feel fluffy, as though the pads are thicker.

PERONEAL NERVE:

At the front of the ankle, a retinaculum holds down the tendons that help the foot to dorsiflex. Behind that retinaculum runs the deep peroneal nerve.

INDICATION: PAIN AND A TENDER SPOT ANTERIOR ANKLE, RESTRICTION IN DORSIFLEXION ON SQUATTING

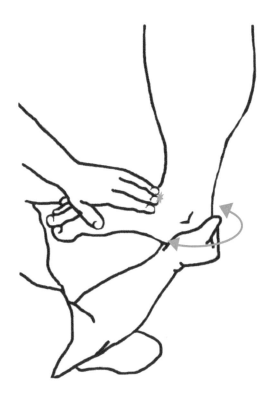

TREATMENT: POSITIONAL RELAXATION APPROACH

1. Patient is sitting on edge of a high treatment table. Therapist sits on low stool. Affected foot sits on therapist's knee. A stool supports the other foot.

2. Find tender point in the anterior ankle crease with one hand. With your knee, bend patient's foot into as much dorsiflexion as possible. Tender point will reduce, but will likely not completely resolve.

3. Place other hand firmly around heel. Carefully twist heel either clockwise or counterclockwise, whichever direction seems to work best for that individual.

4. Add some inversion or eversion to forefoot, using your knee.

5. Wait for tenderness to disappear, or reduce by at least 80%. Then hold about 2 minutes. Bring patient's foot gently out of dorsiflexion and slowly let go.

6. Ask patient to move their foot around in circles, stretch it etc.

7. Ask patient to stand; reassess range, comfort level. They may be able to squat easier, more comfortably, and further.

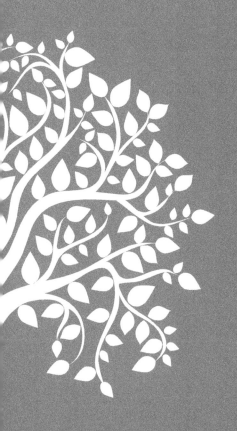

Appendices

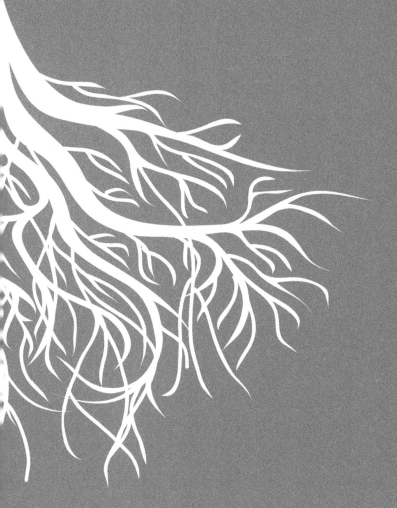

DORSAL RAMI

CUTANEOUS BRANCHES
OF DORSAL ROOT ORIGIN

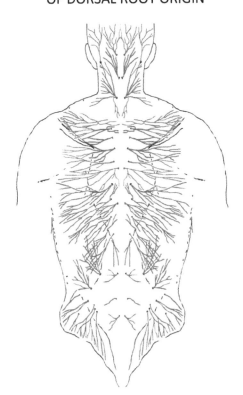

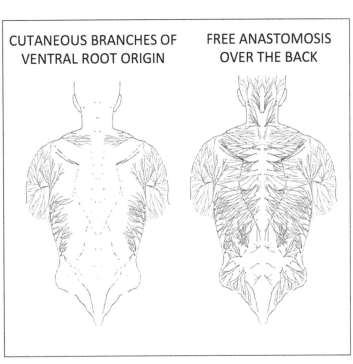

CUTANEOUS BRANCHES OF
VENTRAL ROOT ORIGIN

FREE ANASTOMOSIS
OVER THE BACK

Cutaneous dorsal rami and cutaneous ventral rami freely anastomose over the back.

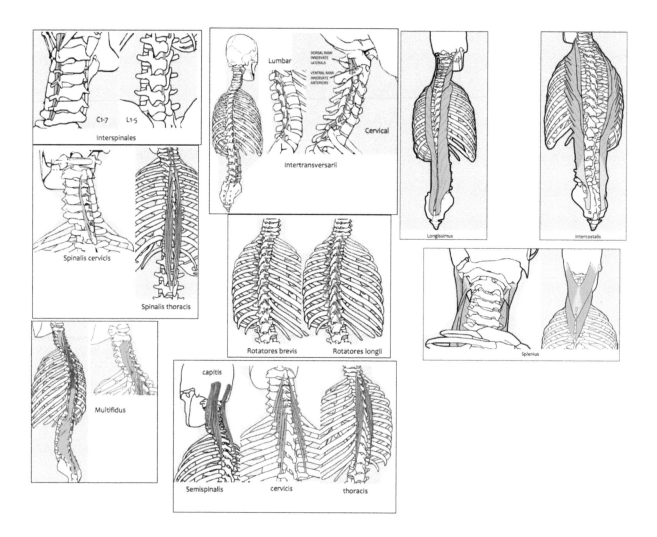

Muscles innervated only by dorsal rami are segmental, and situated behind the transverse processes, buried beneath other muscles that are mainly innervated by ventral rami. Dorsal rami do however, contribute small amounts of motor innervation to all muscles they pierce, close to the spine, on their way to the surface to innervate the skin organ.

VENTRAL RAMI

Cranial Nerves Motor to Neck

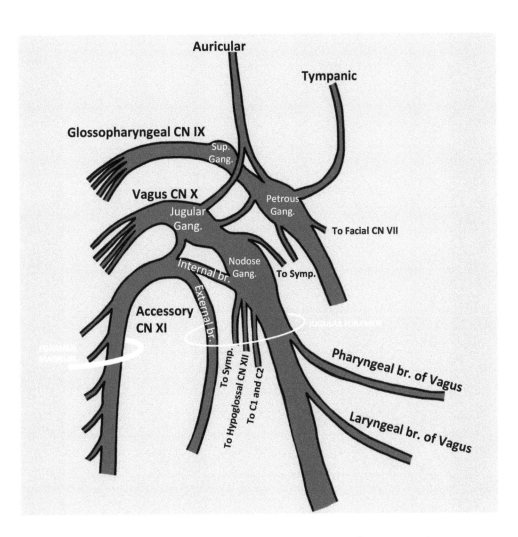

The Accessory nerve CNXI derives from branches of cervical spinal nerves, ascends up into the head through foramen magnum, then descends back out into the periphery through the jugular foramen, along with Vagus nerve CNX and Hypoglossal nerve CN XII.

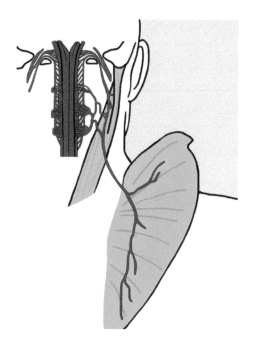

The Accessory nerve innervates sternocleidomastoid and trapezius muscles.

Spinal Nerves Motor to Trunk

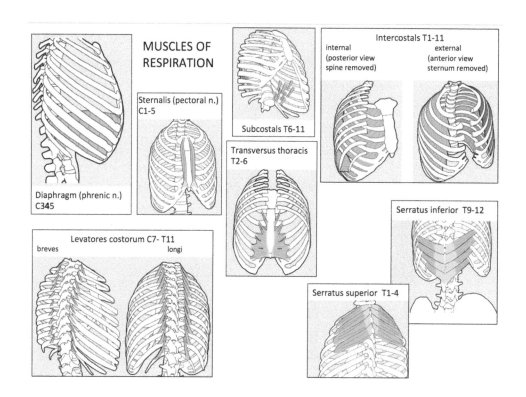

All the muscles involved in respiration that are innervated by spinal nerves.

DermoNeuroModulating | Diane Jacobs

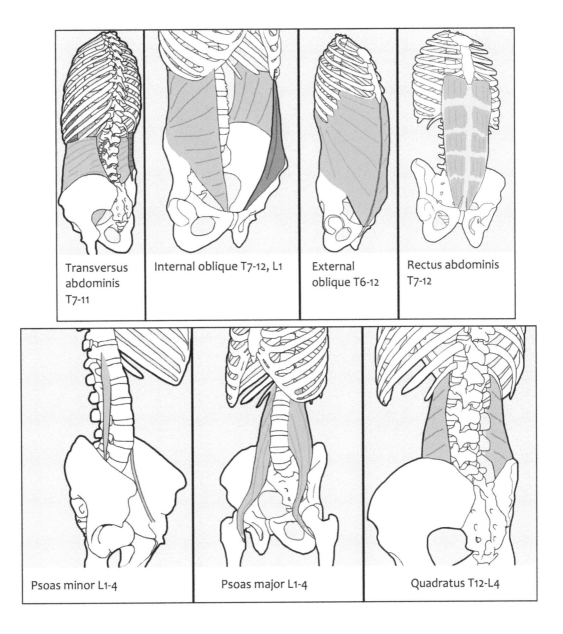

Transversus abdominis T7-11

Internal oblique T7-12, L1

External oblique T6-12

Rectus abdominis T7-12

Psoas minor L1-4

Psoas major L1-4

Quadratus T12-L4

All the muscles of the abdomen and lower trunk that are innervated by spinal nerves.

CERVICAL PLEXUS

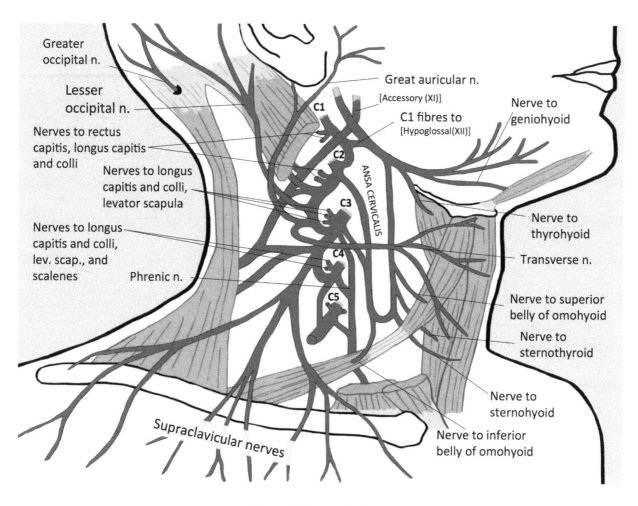

Nerves of the cervical plexus

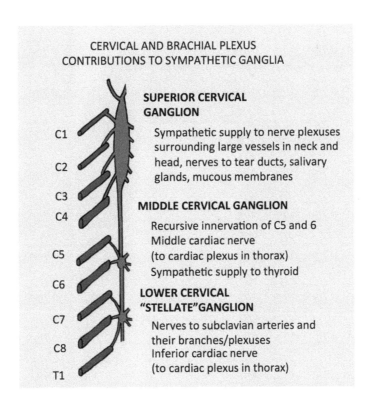

CERVICAL AND BRACHIAL PLEXUS
CONTRIBUTIONS TO SYMPATHETIC GANGLIA

SUPERIOR CERVICAL GANGLION

Sympathetic supply to nerve plexuses surrounding large vessels in neck and head, nerves to tear ducts, salivary glands, mucous membranes

MIDDLE CERVICAL GANGLION

Recursive innervation of C5 and 6
Middle cardiac nerve
(to cardiac plexus in thorax)
Sympathetic supply to thyroid

LOWER CERVICAL "STELLATE" GANGLION

Nerves to subclavian arteries and their branches/plexuses
Inferior cardiac nerve
(to cardiac plexus in thorax)

C1
C2
C3
C4
C5
C6
C7
C8
T1

All the contributions by cervical and brachial plexus to important sympathetic ganglia that serve glands in the head, and form plexuses around major arteries in head, neck and chest, and heart.

NERVES OF CERVICAL PLEXUS

C1 (Motor)
- Contributes to
    - **Hypoglossal n.** (geniohyoid, thyrohyoid)
    - **Vagus (CN X)**
    - **Ansa cervicalis** (superior belly of omohyoid, sternohyoid)
- Forms **Suboccipital nerve**
- **Nerves to** deep neck flexors

C2 (Motor and **Cutaneous**)
- Contributes to
    - **Ansa cervicalis** (omohyoid inferior belly)
    - **Spinal accessory nerve (CN XI)**
- **Nerves to** deep neck flexors
- Contributes to **SUPERFICIAL CERVICAL PLEXUS**
- Forms
    - **TRANSVERSE NERVE**
    - **GREATER AURICULAR**
    - **LESSER OCCIPITAL and GREATER OCCIPTITAL nerves**

C3 (Motor and **Cutaneous**)
- Contributes to **SUPERFICIAL CERVICAL PLEXUS**
- Forms **SUPRACLAVICULAR NERVES**
- **Nerves to** deep neck flexors
- **Nerves to** scalenes
- Contributes to **Ansa cervicalis** (sternothyroid, sternohyoid, omohyoid inferior belly)
- Contributes to **Spinal accessory nerve (CN XI)**

C4 (Motor and **Cutaneous**)
- **Nerves to** deep neck flexors
- Contributes to **Dorsal scapular nerve** and **nerve to** scalenes
- Major supplier of **phrenic nerve** to diaphragm
- Contributes somewhat to **SUPRACLAVICULAR NERVES**
- Contributes to **Spinal accessory nerve (CN XI)**

Summary of cervical plexus nerve destinations.

Summary of Cl nerve root destinations

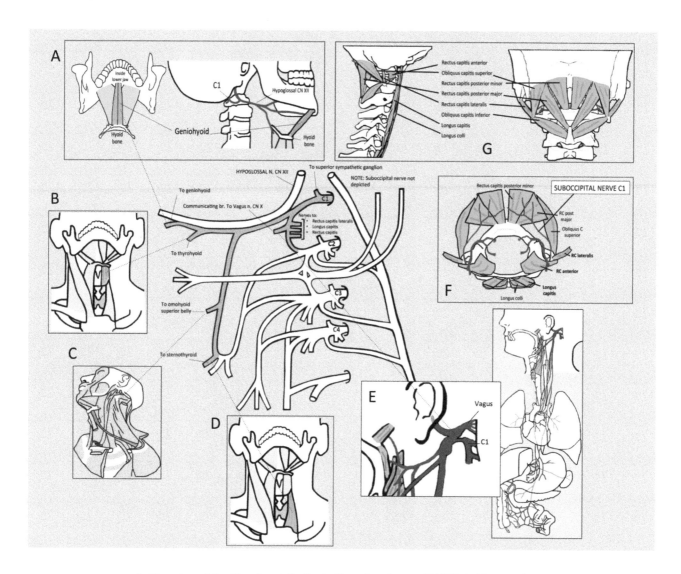

A. Nerve to geniohyoid and contribution to Hypoglossal nerve CN XII; B. Nerve to thyrohyoid; C. Nerve to superior belly omohyoid; D. Nerve to sternohyoid; E. Branch to Vagus CNX; F. Suboccipital nerve; G. Suboccipital nerve supply to suboccipital muscles.

Summary of C2 nerve root destinations

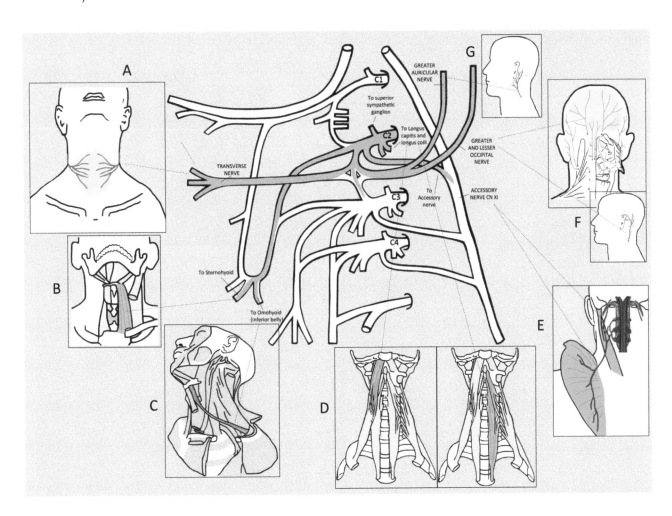

A. Transverse nerve cutaneous to front of neck; B. Nerve to Sternohyoid; C. Nerve to inferior belly of omo-hyoid; D. Segmental contribution to deep neck flexors; E. Segmental contribution to Accessory CN XI; F. Occipital nerves cutaneous to back of head; G. Greater auricular nerve cutaneous to back of head behind ear.

Summary of C3 nerve root destinations

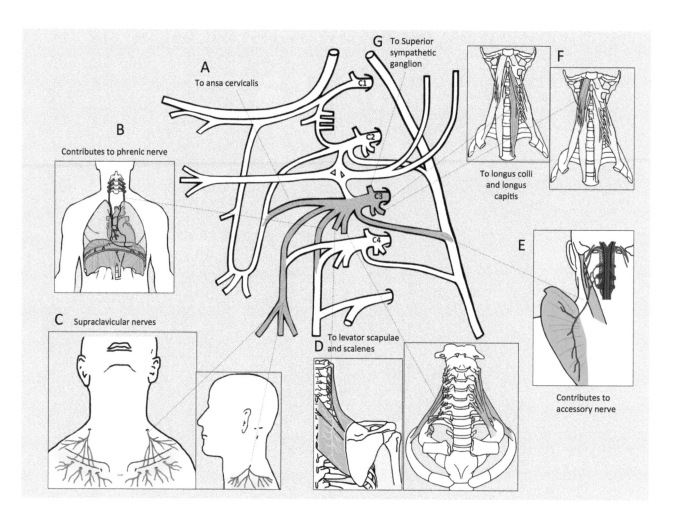

G To Superior sympathetic ganglion

A To ansa cervicalis

B Contributes to phrenic nerve

F To longus colli and longus capitis

C Supraclavicular nerves

D To levator scapulae and scalenes

E Contributes to accessory nerve

A. Contribution to ansa cervicalis; B. Contribution to phrenic nerve; C. Supraclavicular nerves cutaneous to front of chest and shoulders; D. Segmental contribution to nerves to levator scapulae and scalenes; E. Segmental contribution to accessory nerve CN XI; F. Segmental contribution to deep neck flexors.

Summary of C4 nerve root destinations

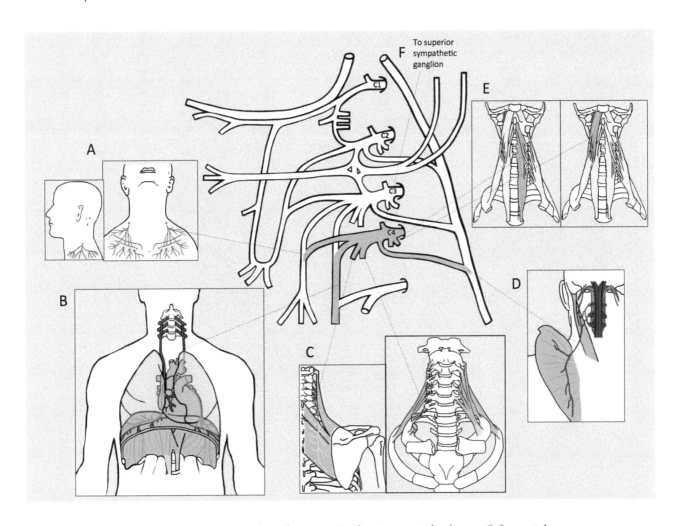

A. Contribution to supraclavicular nerves; B. Phrenic nerve to diaphragm; C. Segmental contribution to levator scapulae and scalenes; D. Segmental contribution to accessory nerve CN XI; E. Segmental contribution to nerves to deep neck flexors.

BRACHIAL PLEXUS

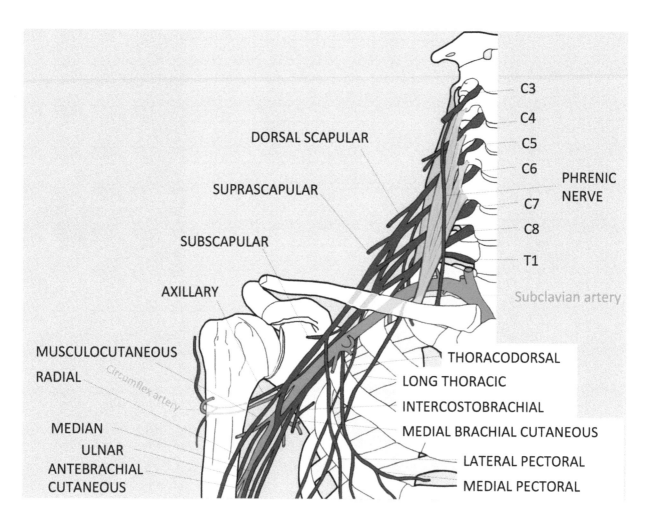

DORSAL SCAPULAR

SUPRASCAPULAR

SUBSCAPULAR

AXILLARY

MUSCULOCUTANEOUS

RADIAL

Circumflex artery

MEDIAN

ULNAR

ANTEBRACHIAL
CUTANEOUS

C3

C4

C5

C6

C7

C8

T1

PHRENIC
NERVE

Subclavian artery

THORACODORSAL

LONG THORACIC

INTERCOSTOBRACHIAL

MEDIAL BRACHIAL CUTANEOUS

LATERAL PECTORAL

MEDIAL PECTORAL

Nerves of the brachial plexus

NERVES FROM THE ROOTS:
1. Dorsal Scapular (C5)
2. Branch to phrenic nerve (C5)
3. Long thoracic nerve (C5,6,7)
4. Branches to longus colli and scalenes (C5,6,7,8)

NERVES FROM THE TRUNKS:
1. Suprascapular (C5,6)
2. Nerve to subclavius (C5,6)

NERVES FROM THE CORDS
1. Lateral pectoral (C5,6,7)
2. Medial pectoral (C8T1)
3. Upper subscapular nerve (C5,6)
4. Middle subscapular (thoracodorsal) (C6,**7,8**)
5. Lower subscapular nerve (C5,6)
6. Medial brachial cutaneous nerve (T1)
7. Medial antebrachial cutaneous nerve (C8T1)

NERVES FROM THE TERMINAL BRANCHES:
1. Musculocutaneous nerve (C5,6,7)
2. Axillary nerve (C5,6)
3. Radial nerve (**C5,6,7,8,**T1)
4. Median nerve (C5,**6,7,8,T1**)
5. Ulnar nerve (C7,**8,T1**)

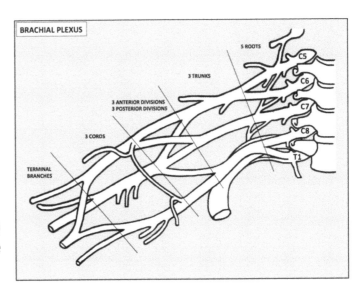

Summary of brachial plexus nerve destinations.

Summary of C5 nerve root destinations

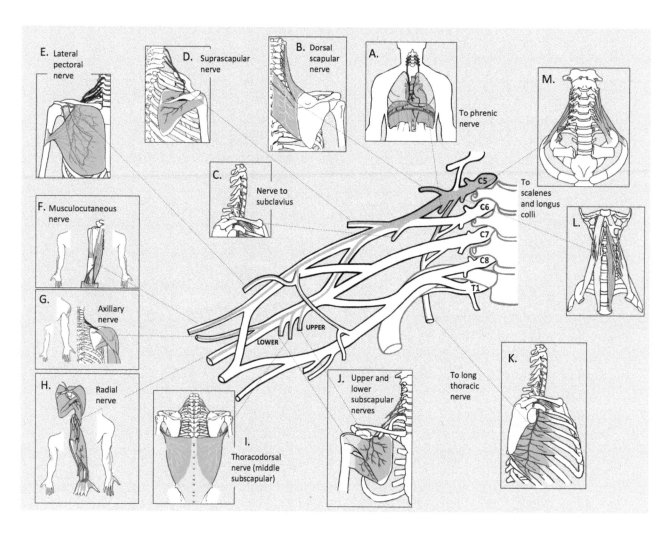

A. Contribution to phrenic nerve; B. Dorsal scapular nerve; C. Nerve to subclavius; D. Suprascapular nerve; E. Lateral pectoral nerve; F. Musculocutaneous nerve; G. Axillary nerve; H. Radial nerve; I. Thoracodorsal nerve (middle subscapular); J. Upper and lower subscapular nerves; K. Contribution to long thoracic nerve; L. Contribution to longus colli; M. Contribution to scalenes

Summary of C6 nerve root destinations

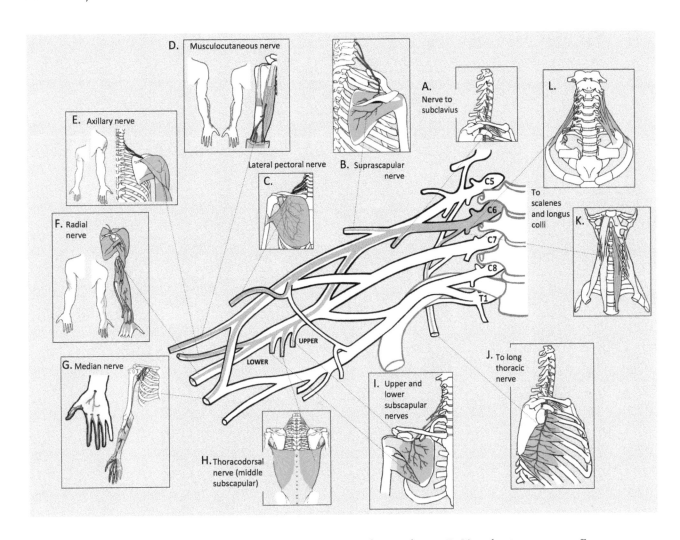

A. Nerve to subclavius; B. Suprascapular nerve; C. Lateral pectoral nerve; D. Musculocutaneous nerve; E. Axillary nerve; F. Radial nerve; G. Median nerve; H. Thoracodorsal nerve (middle subscapular); I. Upper and lower subscapular nerves; J. Contribution to long thoracic nerve; K. nerve to longus colli; L. nerve to scalenes

Summary of C7 nerve root destinations

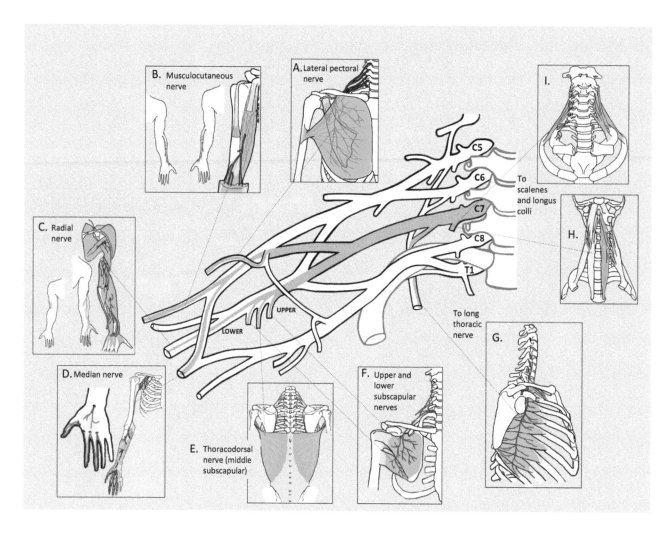

A. Lateral pectoral nerve; B. Musculocutaneous nerve; C. Radial nerve; D. Median nerve;
E. Thoracodorsal nerve (middle subscapular); F. Upper and lower subscapular nerves; G.
Contribution to long thoracic nerve; H. nerve to longus colli; I. Nerve to scalenes

Summary of C8T1 nerve root destinations

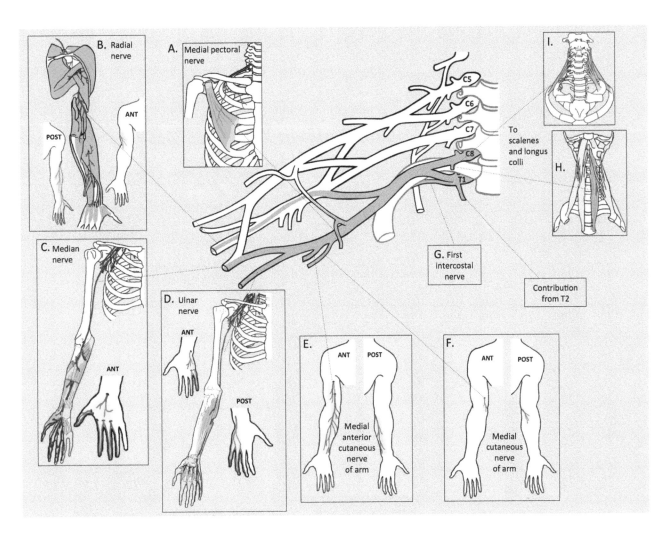

A. Medial pectoral nerve; B. Radial nerve; C. Median nerve; D. Ulnar nerve; E. Medial anterior cutaneous nerve of arm; F. Medial cutaneous nerve of arm; G. First intercostal nerve; H. nerve to longus colli; I. Nerve to scalenes

LUMBAR PLEXUS

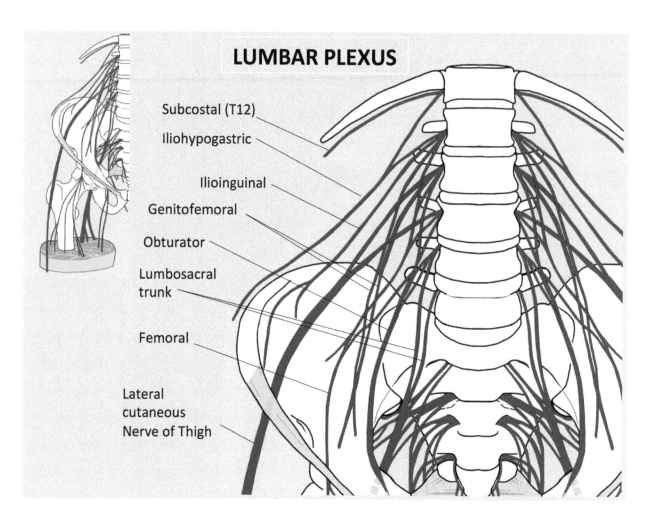

LUMBAR PLEXUS

Subcostal (T12)

Iliohypogastric

Ilioinguinal

Genitofemoral

Obturator

Lumbosacral trunk

Femoral

Lateral cutaneous Nerve of Thigh

Nerves of the lumbar plexus

NERVES OF LUMBAR PLEXUS

L1 (Motor and **cutaneous**)
- Contributes to
    - **Iliohypogastric n** (body wall, skin over lateral pelvis, front of pubis symphysis
    - **Ilioinguinal n** (body wall, skin over upper medial thigh)
    - **Genitofemoral n** (femoral artery, small area of skin over inguinal region, lateral side of genital region, motor for cremaster reflex)
- Forms
    - **Superior cluneal n** (most lateral, supplying skin over buttock)

L2 (Motor and **cutaneous**)
- Contributes to
    - **Genitofemoral n.** (cutaneous to inguinal area, lateral side of testicles [cremaster reflex], supplies femoral artery)
    - **Obturator n.** (supplies hip joint, motor to adductor muscles of thigh, skin of lower inner thigh)
    - **Femoral n.** (motor to knee extensors, cutaneous to medial leg and foot)
    - Motor to psoas and iliacus
- Forms
    - **Lateral cutaneous nerve of thigh**
    - **Middle superior cluneal nerve** (buttock)

L3 (Motor and **cutaneous**)
- Contributes to
    - **Obturator n.** (supplies hip joint, motor to adductor muscles of thigh, skin of lower inner thigh)
    - **Accessory obturator n**
    - **Femoral n.** (motor to knee extensors, cutaneous to medial leg and foot)
    - Motor to psoas and iliacus
    - **Lateral cutaneous nerve of thigh**
    - **Medial superior cluneal nerve** (buttock)

L4 (Motor and **cutaneous**)
- Contributes to
    - **Femoral n.** (motor to knee extensors, cutaneous to medial leg and foot)
    - Motor nerves to psoas and iliacus
    - **Sciatic n.** (motor to all muscles back of thigh, all muscles lower leg and foot, cutaneous to lateral lower leg; top, bottom, outside of foot)
    - **Gluteal n's** (motor to muscles of buttock)

L5 (Motor and **cutaneous**)
- Contributes to
    - **Sciatic n.** (motor to all muscles back of thigh, all muscles lower leg and foot, cutaneous to lateral lower leg; top, bottom, outside of foot)
    - **Gluteal n's** (motor to muscles of buttock)

Summary of lumbar plexus nerve destinations.

Summary of L1 nerve root destinations

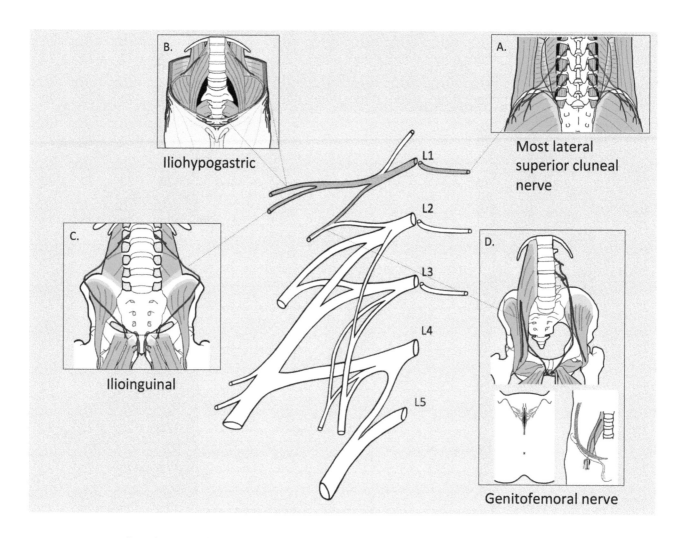

A. Most lateral superior cluneal nerve; B. Iliohypogastric nerve; C. Ilioinguinal nerve; D. Genitofemoral nerve

Summary of L2 nerve root destinations

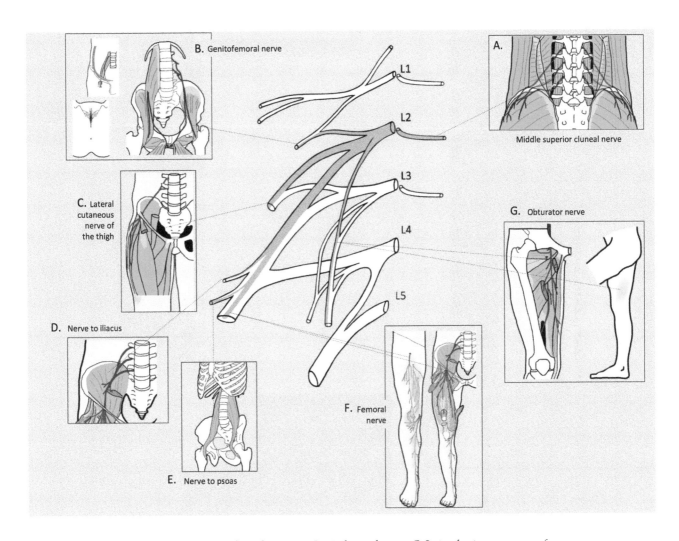

A. Middle superior cluneal nerve; B. Genitofemoral nerve; C. Lateral cutaneous nerve of thigh; D. Nerve to iliacus; E. Nerve to psoas; F. Femoral nerve; G. Obturator nerve

Summary of L3 nerve root destinations

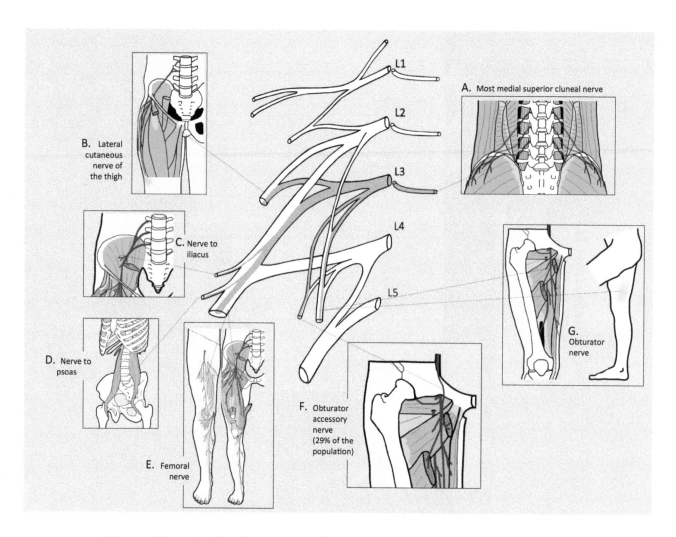

A. Most medial superior cluneal nerve; B. Lateral cutaneous nerve of thigh; C. Nerve to iliacus; D. Nerve to psoas; E. Femoral nerve; F. Obturator accessory nerve (29% of specimens); G. Obturator nerve

Summary of L4 nerve root destinations

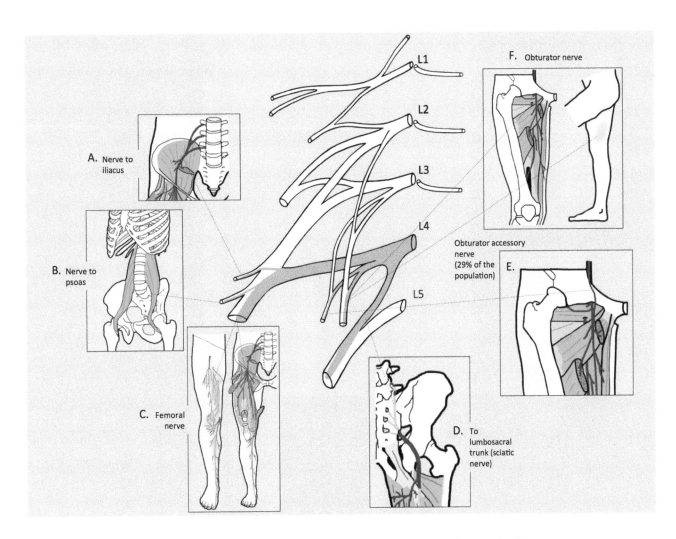

A. Nerve to iliacus; B. Nerve to psoas; C. Femoral nerve; D. Contribution to lumbosacral trunk; E. Obturator accessory nerve (29% of specimens); F. Obturator nerve

SACRAL PLEXUS

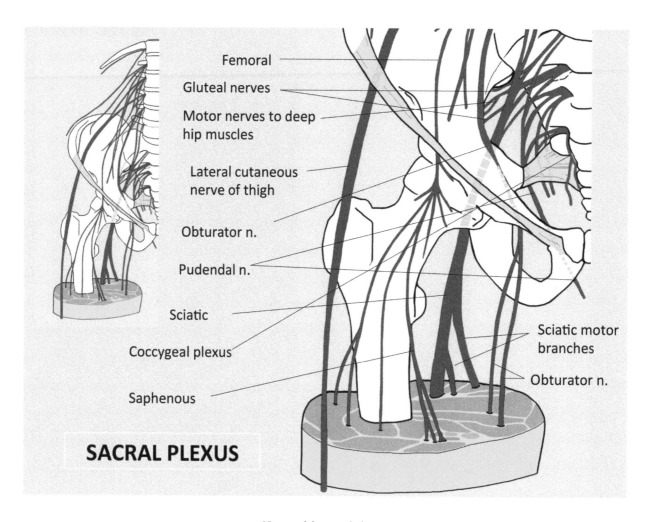

Femoral

Gluteal nerves

Motor nerves to deep hip muscles

Lateral cutaneous nerve of thigh

Obturator n.

Pudendal n.

Sciatic

Coccygeal plexus

Saphenous

Sciatic motor branches

Obturator n.

SACRAL PLEXUS

Nerves of the sacral plexus

NERVES OF SACRAL PLEXUS

S1 (Motor and **cutaneous**)
- Contributes to
    - **Inferior gluteal n.** (motor to muscles of buttock)
    - Motor nerves to quadratus femoris, gemelli, obturator internus
    - **Posterior femoral cutaneous n.**
    - **Sciatic n.**
- Forms
    - **Medial cluneal nerve** (uppermost)

S2 (Motor and **cutaneous**)
- Contributes to
    - **Sciatic n.**
    - Motor nerves to quadratus femoris, gemelli, obturator internus
    - **Posterior femoral cutaneous n. (cutaneous to pelvic floor and back of thigh and leg)**
    - **Perforating cutaneous nerve**
    - **Pudendal n** (motor to pelvic floor smooth and striate muscle, genitalia)
    - Nerves that innervate viscera
- Forms
    - **Middle medial cluneal n.**

S3 (Motor and **cutaneous**)
- Contributes to
    - **Sciatic n**
    - **Posterior femoral cutaneous n**
    - **Perforating cutaneous n.**
    - **Pudendal n.**
    - Nerves to viscera
- Forms
    - most distal **medial cluneal n.**

S4 (Motor and **cutaneous**)
- Contributes to
    - **Sciatic n**
    - **Pudendal n.**
    - Nerves to viscera
    - Nerves to levator ani, anal sphincters
    - **Coccygeal plexus**

S5 (Motor and **cutaneous**)
- Contributes to
    - **Coccygeal plexus** (cutaneous to anus)

Summary of sacral plexus nerve destinations.

Overlap of Lumbar Plexus with Sacral Plexus

Contributions of L4 nerve root to sacral plexus

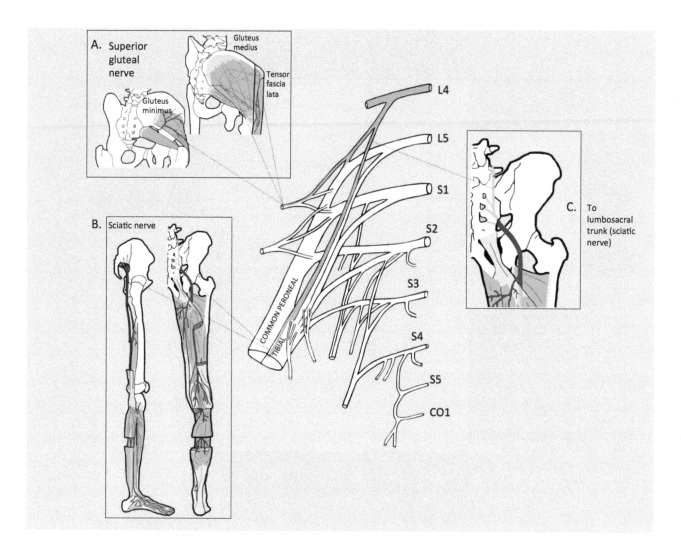

A. Superior gluteal nerve; B. Sciatic nerve; C. Contribution to lumbosacral trunk (sciatic nerve)

Contributions of L5 nerve root to sacral plexus

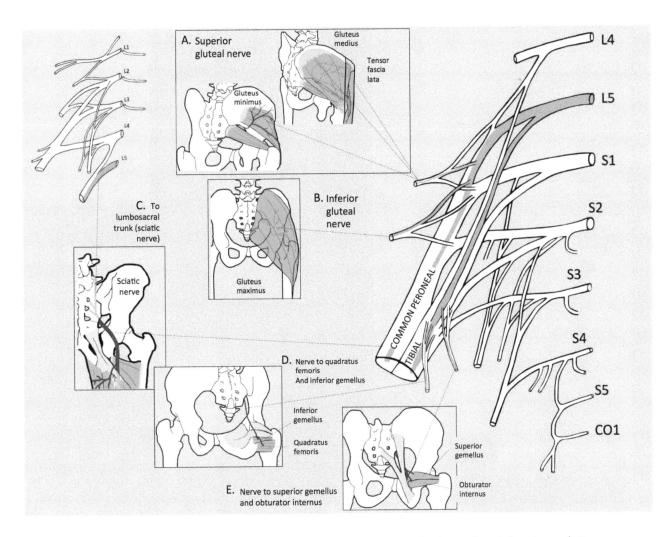

A. Superior gluteal nerve; B. Inferior gluteal nerve; C. Contribution to lumbosacral trunk (sciatic nerve); D. Nerve to quadratus femoris and inferior gemellus; E. Nerve to superior gemellus and obturator internus

Nerves of the Sacral Plexus

Summary of S1 nerve root destinations

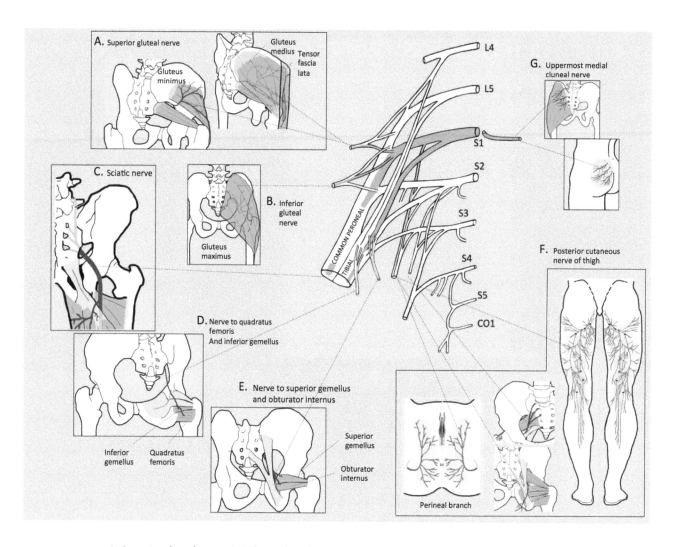

A. Superior gluteal nerve; B. Inferior gluteal nerve; C. Sciatic nerve; D. Nerve to quadratus femoris and inferior gemellus; E. Nerve to superior gemellus and obturator internus; F. Posterior cutaneous nerve of thigh with perineal branch; G. Uppermost medial cluneal nerve

Summary of S2 nerve root destinations

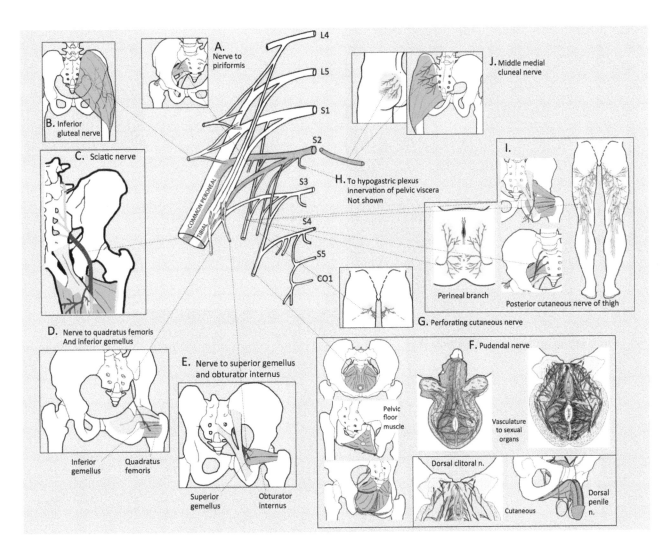

A. Nerve to piriformis; B. Inferior gluteal nerve; C. Sciatic nerve; D. Nerve to quadratus femoris and inferior gemellus; E. Nerve to superior gemellus and obturator internus; F. Pudendal nerve; G. Perforating cutaneous nerve (present in about 29% of specimens); I. Posterior cutaneous nerve of thigh and perineal branch; J. Middle medial cluneal nerve

Summary of S3 nerve root destinations

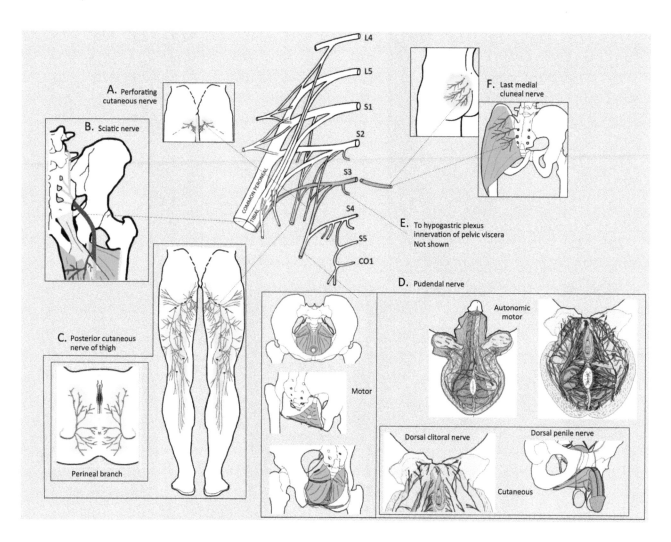

A. Perforating cutaneous nerve; B. Sciatic nerve; C. Posterior cutaneous nerve of thigh with perineal branch;
D. Pudendal nerve; E. Contribution to hypogastric plexus; F. Most caudal of medial cluneal nerves

Summary of S4 nerve root destinations

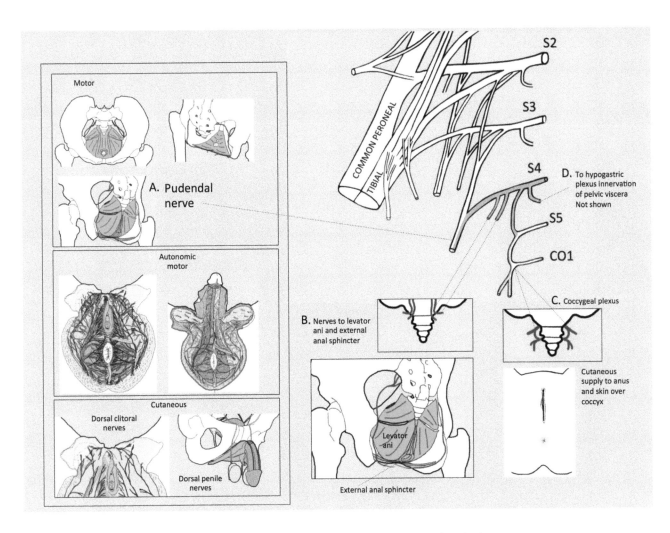

A. Pudendal nerve; B. Nerves to levator ani and external anal sphincter; C. Coccygeal plexus; D. Contribution to hypogastric plexus

Summary of S5, CO1 nerve root destinations

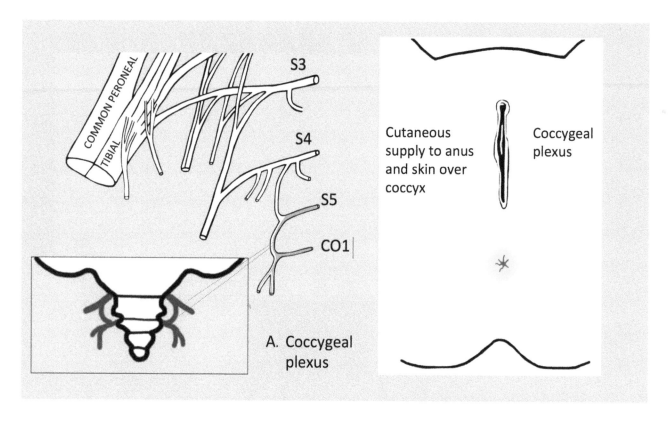

A. Coccygeal plexus

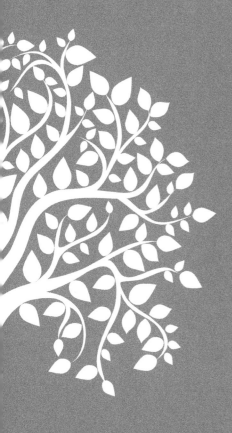

End Chapters

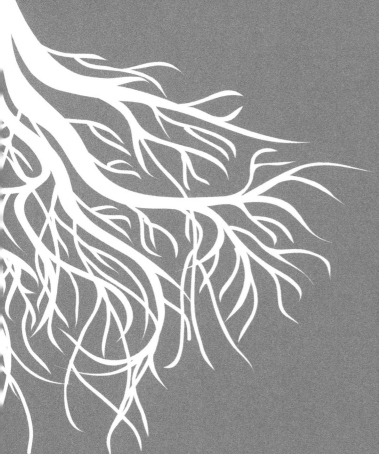

1. A QUICK LOOK AT EVOLUTION OF THE NERVOUS SYSTEM

1. You are a single cell organism. You dominate the planet for billions of years. You do everything through your membrane, the only barrier between you and not-you. You have no nervous system – you do not need one! Your membrane does everything. There are "sensing" pores in it to help you sense your environment. Your membrane moves you about, toward food, away from anything that repels, same way as modern amoebae. You "eat" by wrapping yourself around "food" and engulfing it – yes, right through that membrane which opens up, then closes again. There are "elimination" pores in your membrane to expel your metabolic waste. Congratulations! You have invented all the processes that "life" has to offer: metabolism, excretion, sensitivity, movement, respiration, growth, and reproduction - staving off entropy, by dividing into two fresh cells, is the coolest trick of all!

   (In the human body, we still all start out life as a single cell. Certain cells, such as macrophages in the immune system, and microglia in the brain, still do this pretty basic cell behaviour – they can migrate, and when attracted toward a chemogradient, will move toward it to engulf it.)

2. Fast forward: You are now a multi-cellular organism, so congratulations again! You are a little sea creature that can move around on the sea floor. You are still very small, so most of your cells are surface cells. You now have contractile cells, called "independent effectors" or "myocytes" that contract all by themselves: you still do not have any neurons. Who needs neurons? Not you, not yet, anyway. The environment itself stimulates your myocytes to contract. Your membrane is now a collective membrane, because a membrane operating collectively conserves resources. You can sense through pores in your surface collective membrane, when food is nearby or when danger is nearby, and you can move accordingly,

toward or away from those; not very well, or very fast, but you survive, and life goes on. Until it stops. Because now you can stave off entropy only temporarily, not forever.

You eat by waving tentacles toward your mouth, quite randomly. As generations of you go by however, long skinny body cells develop from sensing pores in the membrane of the tentacles and grow *inward*, and take the sensing pore inside (Ryan and Grant 2009; Myers 2009) *to make contact with the myocytes*. (The sensing pore will later turn into something called a synapse!)

This advance makes it a lot easier to collect food, because these long skinny cells can touch a lot of myocytes at once, and stimulate them all at once! The myocytes can still operate independently, but can also now operate collectively as well! The waving action of your tentacles becomes faster, a lot more coordinated and thus more useful (Swanson 2003).

These neurons are pretty basic. They do both sensing and motor function. The advantage they provide means that creatures that have them will be able to compete successfully and pass them on.

Eventually they make contact with each other within the body and a nerve "net" develops.

(In the human body, we still have a nerve net, represented by our enteric plexus, part of the peripheral nervous system, very autonomous. It is both sensory and motor. It is responsible for business-as-usual movement of food through the digestive tract. Embryologically, our entire nervous system still develops from ectoderm, "outer"-derm, in.)

3. A long time goes by. Now you are larger than the little creature with tentacles. You are now a worm! You have taken on a worm's bilateral body plan. You have twin nerve cords running parallel along both sides of your segmented body. You have ganglia. Everything is interconnected. The neurons have figured out all by themselves, that if they divide up tasks, they can get more stuff done at less cost, thermodynamically. A rudimentary division of labour has begun and an autonomic nervous system communicates to itself and to all body parts. "Decisions" are made in the ganglia. "Feedback" information loops have developed. You and any of the other creatures with these systems thrive and reproduce yourselves.

4. Then one day, you end up with a spinal cord: Congratulations, you are now a fish! You have invented being a vertebrate! At the front end of your spinal cord are little ganglia which now can be called "nuclei." They run all your life processes. You have nociceptive neurons everywhere, especially on the surface to convey "danger" signals. How handy! Your spinal cord is very fast, and coordinates *every*thing, sensory input and motor output. Your spinal cord is pretty basic and reflexive, however it *is* a "*central*" nervous system: It works all by itself, or it can work together with homeostatic front-end nuclei. The front-end nuclei also

work independently to monitor internal organs, or in concert with the spinal cord. You are no longer simply a digestive tube that can move autonomously - you now have dedicated muscles, bones, and so on, that act as levers to help you move about in the water, faster, and a lot of neurons to coordinate all of it. You have a heart that pumps blood around to keep everything going. You burn oxygen! You do not require lungs, however, nor do you have to expend energy to breathe – you can get all the oxygen you need by using that old "absorb it from the environment" strategy, letting water flow over your front end, over cells that have specialized in absorbing oxygen and sharing it around.

Your spinal cord takes over the operation of most of the movement of the body; side-to-side swimming, dodging, and undulating in place using your little fins as rudders. All the muscles in your body are connected to each other, segmentally - your myocytes have differentiated, and a new striped kind has developed for these segmented muscles, which is much easier to coordinate, control, and predict, than those old, smooth-muscle "independent effectors" scattered all over the place ever were. These new, obedient, grouped, striped myocytes will contract beautifully in a rippled, smooth, coordinated manner, if a single neuron asks them to.

(In the human body, we still have much the same kind of spinal cord, which still operates our human version of segmental muscle around the vertebral column, all of which has become buried by muscle that came later. Our spinal cord still has a lively withdrawal reflex, though, which allows it to step in and takes control of all our motor output, should there be any threat such as nociceptive input detected by it. Think of how fast your spinal cord whips your hand off a hot stove burner, long before you even realize it was too hot. Very protective!

There are still "independent effectors" in us, but now they are called "smooth muscle cells." They are plentiful in the skin organ, walls of blood vessels, and in the digestive system where they are coordinated by the enteric plexus. Smooth muscle cells are also found dispersed in fascial sheets. Depending where they are in the body, they are responsive to autonomic motor output, and to substances secreted by nociceptive neurons.

Embryologically, we still start out with gill structures called branchial arches – these develop into other things, however, like jaw and throat structure.)

5. Even more time goes by. You are now a creature who can lug yourself up out of the water onto the riverbank or the sea edge, using lobed fins. You can even breathe for a while outside of water, because you now have sort of a lung organ. Gravity presents quite a challenge though, as your body works best when buoyed up by water. Congratulations! You are Tiktaalik! (Shubin 2009).

6. Eventually, in spite of major obstacles, you remain on land. Evolution goes creative in a big way, giving rise to long lines of animals, some more successful and some less, some huge and some small, some which go back into the water to feed, like sea turtles, some which go back into the water to live, like whales. All the ones who choose to live on land face challenges posed by a whole new environment, and succeed! These include how to deal with gravity and get around, because swimming does not work on land; how to find food; how to stay hydrated; how to avoid becoming somebody else's food; how to mate and reproduce on land; how to stay warm or cool; and myriad other problems to be solved. Limbs evolve, nervous systems enlarge to control them, and sense through them better. Spinal cords remain – they are much too useful and convenient to the organism and all large land species with endoskeletons. Your spinal cord takes on some of the job of moving of your 4 limbs in set patterns, so the front part of your brain can focus more on survival, finding food, raising offspring, and avoiding death by predation. Brains enlarge to more easily coordinate new muscles along longer bones and in faraway digits. Brains and bodies find all sorts of balance points – dinosaurs end up with tiny brains and huge bodies. Along the way, birds, the last dinosaurs, end up with smaller bodies and small, but smart brains. Mammals end up with larger brains, smaller bodies, and the ability to self-thermoregulate.

    You became a mammal – congratulations! You feed your young with specialized sweat glands on the front of your body that make milk. Your enlarged brain *inhibits* a lot of your spinal cord reflexivity, both sensory and motor, so that you have better control of yourself, according to context. Your brain has started to become a bit *predictive*.

7. Goodness, time seems to be going by much quicker. Now you are a primate. Congratulations! You live in a troop. You must remain a member of this troop, for your own protection. You must gain a troop status, or be born into one, and then maintain it. To maintain your place you have to be observant of all the politics going on around you at all times. You must maintain many relationships with many other primates and stay on good terms with them. Your brain has enlarged enough that it can easily cope with all this new social necessity. Social grooming is a fact of life; it is what everybody does when they are not busy finding food or engaging in reproduction or fighting. It coheres and maintains social order. It keeps parasites down (Sapolsky 2007).

8. Oops, what just happened? You are now a human. So, congratulations! Somewhere along the line you became bipedal and learned to cook and make and use weapons and tools. All the primate troop rules still apply; however, now you have a much larger and fancier version of primate brain, three times the size of your nearest modern-day cousin, the chimp. You can choose to remember a lot more, and you can anticipate the future. You can make plans. You can use symbolic thought and language and teach your young how to survive as a socially

dependent human by telling stories, some true, others made-up. You can learn to read and write. You can talk and sing, and invent things. You can mould your environment to suit your needs and wants. You can use your hands to make clothing and art and music and do all sorts of other remarkable things.

Childbirth is no picnic anymore, however (Fischer and Mitteroecker 2015) – brains have enlarged so much that heads have become bigger at birth; babies have to be born in a foetal state in which they are physically helpless, for many months. Nothing can be done about this aspect of the human condition. Pelvic girdle size is a firm evolutionary constraint against any longer gestation time. Your infant brain is extremely dependent, sensitive, and socially, highly malleable. Many of the neurons you are born with die off rapidly. Your human brain does not fully mature until you are about 25 years old, at which time you are left with about 86 billion, highly interconnected neurons (Azevedo et al. 2009). You have become thoroughly and inextricably woven into whatever language and culture you are born into.

Social grooming is still a fact of life. A lot of it has turned to verbal gossip, but it still feels nice when somebody brushes your hair or scratches your back. You will always have neurons that respond to innocuous physical touch, and that inhibit nociception in spinal cord and brain (Foster et al. 2015).

Your culture, including your family of origin and all the experiences you will have as a new human organism with a big brain, learning everything you will come to know and believe, will greatly determine what sort of response your brain develops to deal with noxious input. Mechanisms that evolved biologically within your brain have been conserved, thank goodness, to manage nociceptive input easily and ongoingly most of the time, without you ever having to be aware of any of it. Social stress is probably the biggest danger faced by a biologically intact human nervous system. Social stress can greatly interfere with the production of endogenous opioids made by those old bits of brain, what I like to call the Critterbrain, which we still have along with the earlier spinal cord, or Fishbrain, and which is still much the same as that of all the mammalian quadrupeds in whom it evolved. The Critterbrain is still responsible for everything that has to do with basic life processes and homeostasis and reproductive deployment, and it can end up somewhat disadvantaged in a human brain that matured while undergoing a lot of exogenous social and environmental stressors. Even in a human brain that has successfully matured with optimal amounts of stress that facilitated optimal learning and pathway-building, a noceboic social stress will result in the release of cholecystokinin in the brain, which negates any effects from endogenous opioid production, and can make pain perception worse; furthermore, pain can still arise as if from nowhere, if the Critterbrain stops being able to do its job well for whatever reason.

Now you have a human brain, 5 times larger than other creatures your size (Striedter 2004), with about 86 billion neurons, each one with 10,000 synapses, each synapse managed by 250 million different unique proteins that turn over ever couple of days (Schuman 2013). You have 72 kilometers (45 miles) of peripheral nerves (BodyWorlds 2007), containing evolutionarily conserved neurons that are sensory and autonomic, with sensory neuron cell bodies living in ganglia outside the central nervous system. They have one pole inside the spinal cord, to faithfully report everything they encounter, and together with autonomic efferent neurons, try to manage all output requests from your hierarchical nervous system that mostly ignores them, because it prefers to predict instead.

What if your Critterbrain, for whatever reason, stops suppressing noxious input from the spinal cord? What if it produces a pain experience for no particularly good reason you can see, and you are freaked out about it? You will probably call somebody for some help.

How do we, as *therapists*, get a Critterbrain's *attention*? How can we attempt to get it off whatever square it seems to be stuck on? How can we help the entire nervous system operate more seamlessly again? How can we help more recent nervous system bits dovetail smoothly once again with all the older, more primitive bits, inhibit them, modulate them the way it usually does, effortlessly?

Well, such a brain may well need a safe context and some judiciously applied novel sensory stimuli to pay attention to. We as therapists can provide that. It helps to know what sort of sensory input to provide if we understand what sensory input does, and how it works.

GENERAL FEATURES OF SENSORY INPUT

NOTES: Mostly from C.U.M. Smith's Biology of Sensory Systems, chapter 3 (2008).

1. **All sensory neurons** are classified into mechano-, chemo-, photo-, thermo-. They require *adequate stimulus* – defined as type of stimulus to which a receptor is attuned.

   · All somatosensory neurons have cell bodies in the dorsal root ganglia (or their equivalent within the brain).

   · They all have a terminal pole somewhere in the periphery and a central pole somewhere inside the central nervous system. They do not have dendrites.

   · They are classified into mechano-, chemo-, photo-, thermo-

   · They are either exteroceptive or interoceptive:

   · Monitoring of external environment is important to all living creatures

   · Monitoring of the internal environment is important to brains which must manage thermal homeostasis endogenously

   · They can be of several sizes, from slowly conducting, unmyelinated thin C to fast-conducting, thickly myelinated large A beta type.

   · Nociceptive-capable neurons have a high threshold compared to the rest; they can conduct information that is modality specific or can be poly-modal or wide-dynamic. A subsection of nociceptive capable neurons are thicker, faster and myelinated, the A delta fibres. Most only reach into the CNS as far as the dorsal horn.

2. **"Labeled line"** theory: this pertains to "modality"

   · The biophysics of nerve impulse is identical regardless of fibre type

   · Information from any sense organ is identical to the CNS, so how does it "know" how to interpret whether the signal is sound, light, temperature, odor, except by noting which fiber the info arrives in?

   · Information coming in through the senses is conveyed to appropriate "processing" areas of cortex.

   · Processed information from any and every sensory input is "associated" by the "association" cortex

3. **Intensity:**

   · stimulus intensity is signalled by the *frequency* of action potentials in a sensory nerve fibre of a certain modality (usually many fibres are involved

   · "threshold" is the weakest stimulus that organism can detect

   · thresholds can vary depending on fatigue, context, practice, culture, etc.

   · even with no stimulus, sensory fibres transmit action potentials at a low frequency: this is known as *maintained discharge*

   · CNS has to *learn* to distinguish signal from noise, threshold from maintained, and register "just noticeable difference" described by Weber-Fechner law.

- W-F law describes the relationship between the physical magnitudes of stimuli and the perceived intensity of the stimuli

4. **Adaptation**
   - all non-nociceptive sensory fibres adapt, which means they stop firing after awhile: most nociceptive neurons will continue to fire instead, and are able to sensitize (Woolf 2011). Large A delta nociceptive fibres that respond primarily to thermal stimuli may be able to adapt (Ringkamp et al. 2013, Gebhart et al 2013). (Decrease in perceived pain is likely due to better descending modulation by rostral parts of the CNS, and increase in inhibitory inter-neurons in the spinal cord, than to any decrease of activity by nociceptive-capable neurons.)
   - Processes within the central nervous system, activated by nociceptive input, may further sensitize low-threshold neurons, contributing to more nociceptive input (secondary hyperalgesia, and/or descending facilitation).
   - More rostral areas of the central nervous system must become involved for descending inhibition occur, and raise nociceptive thresholds (Ossipov 2009).

5. **Receptive fields** (RFs):
   - A receptive field is a patch of surroundings the sensory fibre senses; they can be of varying sizes
   - RFs have internal organization – stimulation of one part may lead to sensory excitation and another part, inhibition
   - Very overlapped
   - A trade-off exists between sensory precision and size of RF: for example, sensory neurons in skin of the back have low resolution, low sensory discriminative capacity, and large receptive fields. Sensory neurons in skin over the fingertips have high resolution, precise sensory discriminative capacity, and tiny receptive fields.

6. **Cortical maps of receptive fields**: except for olfactory system, sensory endings and their RFs are arranged in 2-D representational maps:
   - touch receptors of skin -> somatotopic
   - cochlea -> tonotopic
   - retina -> retinotopic
   - Interoceptive neurons (including those with nociceptive capability) are represented by mapping in the insular cortex (Craig 2014).

7. **Hierarchical and parallel function**: several maps interlink and interact with each other with information flow both forward and backward – "tangled hierarchy"; "heterarchy"

8. **Feature extraction and trigger stimuli**: ever more specific features of the sensory world are 'extracted' as sensory info flows forward through the brain
   - These will be the features ***important to the creature sensing them.***

REFERENCES

1. Ryan, T.J. and Grant, S.G.N., 2009, The origin and evolution of synapses. Nat Rev Neurosci. Oct;10(10):701-12.

2. Myers, P.Z., 2009, The ubiquity of exaptation. Pharyngula blog Dec. http://scienceblogs.com/pharyngula/2009/12/05/the-ubiquity-of-exaptation/

3. Swanson, L.W., (Author), 2003, Brain Architecture: Understanding the Basic Plan. Oxford University Press

4. Shubin, N., (Author), 2009, Your Inner Fish. Vintage; Revised ed. edition Jan 6.

5. Sapolsky, R., (Author), 2007, A Primate's Memoir: A Neuroscientists's Unconventional Life Among the Baboons. Simon and Schuster, Nov 1

6. Fischer, B., and Mitteroecker, P., 2015, Covariation between human pelvis shape, stature, and head size alleviates the obstetric dilemma. Proc Natl Acad Sci U S A. , May 5; 112(18): 5655–5660.

7. Azevedo, F.A., Carvalho, L.R., Grinberg, L.T., Farfel, J.M., Ferretti, R.E., Leite, R.E., Jacob-Filho, W., Lent, R., and Herculano-Houzel, S., 2009, Equal numbers of neuronal and nonneuronal cells make the human brain an isometrically scaled-up primate brain. J Comp Neurol. Apr 10;513(5):532-41

8. Foster, E., Wildner, H., Tudeau, L., Haueter, S., Ralvenius ,W.T., Jegen, M., Johannssen, H., Hösli, L., Haenraets, K., Ghanem, A., Conzelmann, K., Bösl, M., and Zeilhofer, H.U., 2015, Targeted Ablation, Silencing, and Activation Establish Glycinergic Dorsal Horn Neurons as Key Components of a Spinal Gate for Pain and Itch. *Neuron*, Mar. 85: 1289-1304

9. Striedter, G.F. (Author), 2004, Principles of Brain Evolution. Sinauer Associates Inc Oct. 30

10. Schuman, E., 2013, The Remarkable Neuron: Erin Schuman at TEDxCaltech. Feb 8. https://www.youtube.com/watch?v=yr6kh_QOk0s

11. BodyWorlds Exhibit, 2007, Science World, Vancouver, B.C.

12. Smith, C.U.M. (Author), 2008, Biology of Sensory Systems. Chapter 3 pp31-39, published online Nov. 24.

13. Woolf, C.J., 2011, Central sensitization: implications for the diagnosis and treatment of pain. Pain. Mar., 152(3 Suppl): S2-15

14. Ringkamp M, Raja SN, Campbell JN, Meyer RA. Peripheral mechanisms of cutaneous nociception. In: Textbook of Pain (6th ed.), edited by McMahon SB, Koltzenburg M, Tracey I, Turk DC, editors. Philadelphia, PA: Elsevier: 2013, p. 1–30.

15. Gebhart, G.F., Schmidt, Robert F. (Eds.), 2013, Encyclopedia of Pain; Ringkamp, M., and Meyer, R.A., Nociceptor, Adaptation. Reference Work Entry, Encyclopedia of Pain. Pp 2232-2233. http://link.springer.com/referenceworkentry/10.1007%2F978-3-642-28753-4_2782

16. Ossipov M.H., (Author of chapter), 2009, Pain Pathways: Descending Modulation. Ed. Larry R Squire; Encyclopedia of Neuroscience, Elsevier Ltd

17. Craig, A.D (Bud) (Author), 2014, How Do You Feel? An Interoceptive Moment with your Neurobiological Self. Princeton University Press Dec. 21

2. PAIN IS IN THE NERVOUS SYSTEM

There are all sorts of definitions for pain, but we will start with the official one from the International Association for the Study of Pain (IASP):

> *"An unpleasant sensory and emotional experience associated with actual or potential tissue damage, or described in terms of such damage."* - http://www.iasp-pain.org/ Taxonomy#Pain

The word "potential" in this definition suggests to us that pain is not irrevocably correlated to tissue damage, rather to "danger," and to the brain's own opinion about the state of its body.

When we experience pain, it is *we* for whom the experience is unpleasant, sensory, and emotional. Our predictive brains do not particularly care what "we" experience, which might be "pain"; they just do their own work, filtering input, in the moment, from a large number of sources, including whatever experiences we have had through a lifetime, the current context they are in, and ongoing sensory input, to decide what current reality is. Our spinal cords simply do not care; their job is to reflexively protect and guard. If you touch a hot surface like the burner of a stove, by accident, your spinal cord will detect "danger" and will pull your hand off that stove faster than the nociceptive information can even reach your brain to be experienced as "painful."

> *"Before discussing the anatomical and physiological bases for the generation of pain, it is important to reiterate the difference between nociception and pain. Nociception refers to the peripheral and central nervous system (CNS) processing of information about the internal or external environment, as generated by the activation of nociceptors. Typically, noxious stimuli, including tissue injury, activate nociceptors that are present in peripheral structures and that transmit information to the spinal cord dorsal horn or its trigeminal homologue,*

Dermoneuromodulation | Diane Jacobs

the nucleus caudalis. From there, the information continues to the brainstem and ultimately the cerebral cortex, where the perception of pain is generated. Pain is a product of higher brain center processing, whereas nociception can occur in the absence of pain."

- From Chapter 2, Mechanisms of Pain (online), National Research Council (US) Committee on Recognition and Alleviation of Pain in Laboratory Animals, 2009

Let us briefly track how pain has been regarded in the past.

BOTTOM UP, LABELLED LINE

When René Descartes (1596-1650) finally made space for science to enter the human sphere, pain was regarded a specific sense or input *to* the brain *from* the body. I think it is fair to say that the entire subsequent biomedical model of pain was built and has rested ever since, on this premise. I think it is fair to say that this model still implies that anyone who experiences pain without any recent tissue damage is considered, by default, to be "somatising" psychological distress. I think it is fair to say that this divide between mind and body sums up "Cartesian dualism."

GATE THEORY

In 1965, Melzack and Wall published a pivotal paper outlining their now famous gate theory of pain, "Pain Mechanisms, A New Theory," (1965). Briefly, it countered the prevailing biomedical model and its preferred specificity theory for pain, and proposed instead, that within the spinal cord a gating mechanism for pain might exist.

The paper made the biomedical community think, and think hard. In 1973 the International Association for the Study of Pain was launched by John Bonica, chair of the Department of Anaesthesiology at the University of Washington in Seattle (Jones 2010). Ronald Melzack was a presenter. Arrangements were made to publish the journal, PAIN. Patrick Wall was named editor-in-chief. It has steadily grown over decades, with an international conference held every two years attended by thousands of delegates.

Fast-forward 50 years from Melzack and Wall's paper: just last year, Foster and colleagues (Foster et al 2015) provided the first *direct* evidence to support the gate theory of pain: large sensory fibres stimulate inhibitory interneurons in the spinal cord that decrease input from nociceptors. This is the *only solid* evidence so far, for us as manual therapists, that touching people in pain in a kind, non-nociceptive manner might be a good idea, *physically, in a bottom-up way, physiologically,* as well as top-down, psychosocially.

BIOPSYCHOSOCIAL MODEL

George Engel (1977) described in detail how the biomedical model, in its insistence on maintaining Cartesian mind-body dualism, put his field of psychiatry in a very unenviable position; he questioned the definition of "disease," and called for the adoption of a more reality-based model for medicine that he called a biopsychosocial model of illness.

Pain science seems to be more appropriately framed by Engel's biopsychosocial model more than by a strictly biomedical model nowadays.

In some physical therapy circles, the idea of a socio-psycho-bio model of pain has been informally discussed.

Quintner et al. (2008) critiqued the biopsychosocial model as it pertains to pain, proposing that pain is best viewed as an "aporia," "a mystery, a space to which we are denied access" (p 829). Both practitioner and patient, however, can access an "intersubjective third space, from which new therapeutic possibilities can arise." The authors compared the nervous systems of practitioner and patient to musicians creating jazz improvisation, listening to each other and building upon each other's give and take (p 832).

I doubt there could be a better metaphor for what goes on all the time, wordlessly or with accompanying words, during careful manual therapy.

WITHDRAWAL REFLEX

In Netter's Atlas of Neuroscience 2003 is a lovely sequence of images depicting all the various reflexes that occur in the spinal cord, as well as all the bits of nervous system that affect primary synapses there, by interneurons, or by neurons descending from the brain.

One image in particular intrigued me – the withdrawal reflex, which is strictly a spinal cord mediated motor output in vertebrates (Felton 2003).

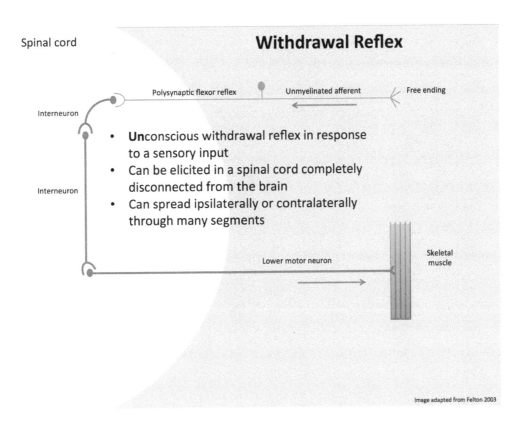

Note the sentence, "Can be elicited in a spinal cord completely severed from the brain."

In a quite creepy video on you tube, which is fascinating once you get past the creepiness factor, a woman tries to skin a fish that has been decapitated and eviscerated. No brain. No guts. Empty, cleaned fish, sliced all the way down the front. It lies inert on the cutting board (Cupp 2014).

As soon as she picks it up by the tail with a towel, so that she can get a grip, and tries to scrape off its scales with a knife, it twists and fights and tries to get away.

That reflex is alive and well and probably operating as hard as it can, in every human spinal cord in anyone who has pain, in every human spinal cord that has undergone cellular changes that have enhanced nociceptive input. Any nociceptive input from the body (but for that involving the face or teeth) is first handled by the spinal cord. The more the spinal cord tries to be protective by deploying its withdrawal reflex, the worse the situation may become for peripheral nerves: The last thing they (or any of their attached vessels) need is yet more compression or tensioning. They need movement, *yes* – but not unconscious, spinal cord-deployed chronic, tonic muscle contraction squeezing and pulling on them.

When you have someone lie down, horizontally, a lot of surface area now supported by a treatment table or floor, there is no way that the nervous system as a whole should feel obliged to keep muscle in tonic contraction. So, if you reach behind the recumbent patient to palpate their back, and feel rigid pipe-like hardness off to one or both sides of the spinous processes, you might plausibly conclude that the spinal cord is not being sufficiently inhibited, and is responding to a constant dribble of nociceptive input. Not from you, because you are not pressing hard enough to elicit any nociception - rather, tonically, over time, it may be reacting to below-the-patient's-awareness-threshold nociceptive input from some nerve or nerves, at *any* distance from their entry/exit place at the spine. Moreover, spinal muscles are not the only muscles the spinal cord may commandeer - it can plausibly interfere with normal movement or muscle extensibility in *any* part of the body below the chin and back of the head.

We can, I think, regard the spinal cord as the oldest, bossiest, most reflexive, most physically protective portion of the central nervous system, ever present and ready and able to commandeer the motor output system to withdraw reflexively in response to danger signals in all vertebrates, regardless of how large our brains may have become. I think it behooves us, therefore, to not make our patients' brains have to work any harder to inhibit spinal cord processing by deliberately activating *more* nociception, because of some (possibly misleading) idea that it should help: I think such approaches may dissociate people from their own nervous systems even more, instead of creating a context in which they might re-inhabit them, seamlessly and effortlessly. A manual therapist can treat people just fine *without* hurting them. That is what this book is about.

DESCENDING MODULATION

Studies of animals and humans show that "pain" is pretty much entirely context dependent. In many animals (and us too probably, but maybe not all of us), in the face of a physical attack a stress response occurs: the periaqueductal grey (PAG) region of the hindbrain deploys either a "fight or flight" response or a "faint and get ready to die" response (Satpute et al. 2013).

Imagine this: you are a wildebeest or some other grazing animal, peacefully minding your own business. A lion jumps out of the grass and onto your back. Your stress response kicks in. Your Critterbrain takes over movement. Your survival mechanisms come on full force.

In the fight/flight response, the main substance secreted in the brain and spinal cord, is noradrenalin from locus ceruleus and other brainstem nuclei, which will make you not care about "pain" – i.e., you may be getting scratched, clawed, bitten with all the nociceptive input that goes with it, but you will not notice - or if you do, you will not care. Your sympathetic nervous system will be turned on full blast. The dorsolateral part of your PAG will be active. Heart rate will go up. Pupils will enlarge, all the better to see the world through. Digestion will shut down - the grass you just ate will sit still for a while. Blood will shunt rapidly away from your entire skin organ, into the muscle layer of the body, adding volume, which will "pump up" muscle to add amazing power to your physical effort to move. You are in the fight of your life, dammit! - you are not ready to just sit there and become somebody else's lunch.

Think about it: Blood pressure will go up. Body compartments containing *striped* muscle fill with extra blood; muscles engorge and become better levers. Digestion halts for awhile, as it would be a waste of energy in a moment of crisis. The skin organ around the body, which accounts for about 8%

of the weight of the body, and contains 10 times more blood reserve than it needs for its own metabolism (Standring 2008) will turn into a much lighter and much looser protective shell, able to stretch much further. Handy if you have long predator teeth buried in your fatty cervico-thoracic hump! They will be biting down into something that has suddenly become slidier around the body, so when you twist and buck to dislodge the lion, the unpredictable ballistic forces you generate, with all those lovely engorged, pumped muscles inside a tough fascial containment membrane with blood that is delivering way more oxygen and glucose than normal to every fibre, might just mean that you will be able to whip that lion right off your back, keep it from reaching front or sides of your vulnerable neck. Plus, the lack of blood flow to the outer skin organ layer, just then, means that much less of that particular precious substance will be lost to the environment. (Really, when you stop to think about it, it is no wonder that our nervous system evolved to not have much sensory-discriminative capacity in the skin of the back.)

What if you lose the fight? There is an alternative stress response available, just in case: the "faint and get ready to die" brain strategy involves the more ventrolateral part of the PAG (Bandler and Shipley 1994). In this response, opioids are secreted. Heart rate slows. Pupils shrink. The animal gives up and keels over, goes unconscious. One hopes it feels no pain, as it becomes a meal for the other creature.

Or maybe it will not, not today! Possums have perfected this strategy successfully to the point where "faint and play dead" seems to be the only one they use anymore. Most of the time, it seems, predators become less interested in prey that no longer moves, if they did not directly kill it, and if they do not feel hungry enough to eat something that seems dead. Thus do animals survive sometimes, and thus did the mechanism evolve to be conserved as a nervous system response that is hard wired.

SUMMARY

Context-sensitive nuclei in the core of the brain make a wide variety of biomolecules (such as noradrenaline, opioids, serotonin) that descend through the spinal cord to gate nociceptive input, or enhance it, depending on circumstance and context (Ossipov 2009, Ossipov et al. 2014). Butler (2013) calls these nuclei "the drug cabinet in the brain."

Thank you, evolution.

NEUROMATRIX FRAMEWORK

By far the bulk of evidence that supports our hands-on work is the top-down kind, psychosocial more than bio. In 2001 Ronald Melzack published a paper (Melzack 2001) on his neuromatrix framework for pain, which he had developed over previous decades. In their 2013 paper, titled simply "Pain," Ronald Melzack and Joel Katz provide a succinct history of the study of pain and of the various conceptual frameworks for it that rose and fell over the centuries.

"Pain is a personal, subjective experience influenced by cultural learning, the meaning of the situation, attention, and other psychological variables. Pain processes do not begin with the stimulation of receptors. Rather, injury or disease produces neural signals that enter an active nervous system that (in the adult organism) is the substrate of past experience, culture, and a host of other environmental and personal factors. These brain processes actively participate in the selection, abstraction, and synthesis of information from the total sensory input. Pain is not simply the end product of a linear sensory transmission system; it is a dynamic process that involves continuous interactions among complex ascending and descending systems." ~ From the abstract, Pain (2013), by Melzack and Katz.

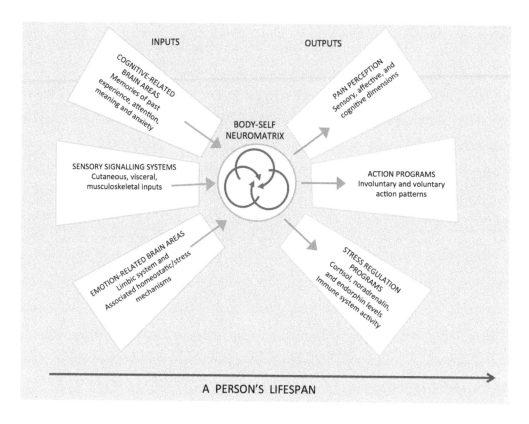

Adapted from Melzack's Neuromatrix diagram

This means that we must be contextual architects (Blickenstaff 2011), first and foremost. This means that we as practitioners, enter into, and become part of that "dynamic process" involving "continuous interactions among complex ascending and descending systems." (Melzack and Katz 2013). Our patients' brains map *us* and any novel input, verbal or otherwise, that we have to offer, right in along with all the other activity they conduct, constantly. They will then choose to either exploit it or ignore it. We do not have any control over, or steerage of that process; all we can do is avoid adding any more nocebo or nociceptive load.

"Words are neurological events. They are meaning-laden puffs of air that our brain transforms into knowledge, opinions, emotions or danger signals." ~Michael Vagg, 2015

Pain cannot be measured; only pain *behaviour* (an output) can be measured. When people tell you about their pain, describe it, this is also pain behaviour.

Pain is a protective response constructed by a brain within an organism, e.g., human, with a life history. A nervous system detects a threat to itself, conscious or unconscious, from without or within, perhaps in the form of some runaway, physiological, positive feedback loop, and forwards it to conscious awareness. By the time pain is perceived by conscious awareness it has already been filtered through all previous experience and behaviour. It is perceived by one's conscious awareness *as though* it were coming from the body. Consciousness is involved; no one has ever managed to define exactly what that means, either.

"We like to think our senses can give us unbiased, truthful information about the external world.... that's utter nonsense - we are not driving the bus. By the time we are aware of a sensation, that sensation has already been filtered and edited and combined with our expectations and our emotions and our personal history so in the end there is no sensation without emotion, there is no sensation without personal history without evolutionary history - it's all combined into a mush and that's what we have to deal with." ~ David J. Linden

"The account of perception that's starting to emerge is what we might call the "brain's best guess" theory of perception: perception is the brain's best guess about what is happening in the outside world. The mind integrates scattered, weak, rudimentary signals from a variety of sensory channels, information from past experiences, and hard-wired processes, and produces a sensory experience full of brain-provided color, sound, texture, and meaning. We see a friendly yellow Labrador bounding behind a picket fence not because that is the transmission we receive but because this is the perception our weaver-brain assembles as its best hypothesis of what is out there from the slivers of information we get. Perception is inference." ~ Atul Gwande, in "The Itch," 2008

"At first glance, pain seems relatively straightforward – hitting one's thumb with a hammer hurts one's thumb. Such experiences are easily understood with a structural-pathology model, which supposes pain provides an accurate indication of the state of the tissues. However, on closer inspection, pain is less straightforward. Much of the pain we see clinically fits into this less straightforward category, where pain cannot be understood as a marker of the state of the tissues. This paper argues that the biology of pain is never really straightforward, even when it appears to be. There are four key points:

- *that pain does not provide a measure of the state of the tissues;*
- *that pain is modulated by many factors from across somatic, psychological and social domains;*
- *that the relationship between pain and the state of the tissues becomes less predictable as pain persists; and*
- *that pain can be conceptualised as a conscious correlate of the implicit perception that tissue is in danger."*

~ Lorimer Moseley, Reconceptualising Pain According to Modern Pain Science. BodyinMind blog, retrieved May 7 2016

Various patterns of brain activity, imaged while subjects received painful stimuli, have been referred to as "pain systems" or "pain networks" or "the pain matrix" in the brain, **in**correctly, according to Legrain et al. who argued against this idea (Legrain et al. 2011). They said (paraphrased), the same network activates with any sort of looming stimulus that looks threatening. Therefore it should be called a salience network, not a pain matrix. If a wasp comes close and looks dangerous, you will reach out to swat the wasp before it can sting - the exact same network activates in the absence of any actual nociceptive input!

Their conclusion is supported by evidence stemming from rubber hand illusions, wherein the subject's sense of "self" is induced to incorporate a visible rubber hand, by stroking the skin on the (hidden) real hand, and the rubber hand, simultaneously: once the illusion is established, the operator strikes the rubber hand with a hammer (BBC Two 2010). The subject's dismay is immediate and evident.

PHILOSOPHICAL CONSIDERATIONS

PHENOMENOLOGY

Pain *is* a real problem, but it is an experience, generated within the nervous system, and it is wholly, entirely subjective:

> *"Phenomenology is the study of structures of consciousness as experienced from the first-person point of view. The central structure of an experience is its intentionality, its being directed toward something, as it is an experience of or about some object."* -

- Stanford Encyclopedia of Philosophy online

If pain is, in this case, an 'object' that someone is (subjectively) 'experiencing', or about which someone is distressed, phenomenology makes a great deal of sense as philosophical underpinning. Even though pain is subjective, to the person who has it, it *can* feel like a real "object" – in particular it can feel like a physical obstacle to movement, as can the body part in which pain is experienced as having arisen.

EMBODIED COGNITION

"Cognition is embodied when it is deeply dependent upon features of the physical body of an agent, that is, when aspects of the agent's body beyond the brain play a significant causal or physically constitutive role in cognitive processing."

- Stanford Encyclopedia of Philosophy online

May we presume, by "aspects of the agent's body" they mean peripheral neurons? It is not exactly clear. They could be referring to all sorts of non-neuronal aspects. Which to me (and I could be wrong) makes no particular sense, in terms of the word, "cognition." Yes, sunflower stems (a nod to Varela and Maturana 1980, who were the originators of this idea, apparently) can twist to track the sun across the sky – but are they "cognizing"? *Really?* Were the "independent effectors," the freely contracting myocytes discussed earlier, in small, non-neuronal multi-cell sea creatures, able to "cognize"? Can any single-cell organism "cognize"?

Within the PT profession, mostly in Europe, there has been an effort to find better philosophical underpinnings than Descartes, and lessen dualism inherent in the biomedical model. "Embodied cognition" has been getting a lot of buzz in such circles.

THE BRAIN IS PREDICTIVE, NOT REACTIVE

It takes account of everything, and then ignores most of it. It exhibits hierarchical functions, which means it is great at ignoring and inhibiting sensory input and feedback it regards as inconsequential. It exhibits parallel functions, which means that its representational maps interlink and interact with each other both forward and backward within the sensory stream (Smith 2008). It uses feature extraction when triggered by a stimulus, which means that ever more specific features of the sensory world are 'extracted' as sensory info flows forward through the brain, and these will be the features *important to the creature sensing them* - in our case, human creatures (Smith 2008).

a. To a large extent we can influence our patients into paying attention to whatever we *think* (as therapists) they should pay attention to during treatment and between treatments.

b. This is a *professional responsibility*: we owe it to our patients to not distract them with meaningless observations or concepts, which could be harmful by being noceboic. We owe them the service of helping them to come into improved relationship with their own nervous systems, of which they are the conscious, self-aware social-seeking part.

Your brain is predictive, not reactive. For many years, scientists believed that your neurons spend most of their time dormant and wake up only when stimulated by some sight or sound in the world. Now we know that all your neurons are firing constantly, stimulating one another at various rates. This intrinsic brain activity is one of the great recent discoveries in neuroscience. Even more compelling is what this brain activity represents: millions of predictions of what you will encounter next in the world, based on your lifetime of past experience. ~ Lisa Feldman Barrett, answering the 2016 Edge.org question, "What do you consider the most interesting recent [scientific] news? What makes it important?"

"The short punch line of this book is that brains are foretelling devices and their predictive powers emerge from the various rhythms they perpetually generate. At the same time, brain activity can be tuned to become an ideal observer of the environment, due to an organized *system* of rhythms." ~ György Buzsáki, Rhythms of the Brain 2008.

EMBODIED PREDICTION

I much prefer this term as opposed to embodied "cognition." (Clark 2013). It makes a lot more sense to me. Neurons evolved from the outside in. Neurons and nervous systems in us *still* develop from ectoderm ('outer' derm) (Swanson 2003).

Before there was central nervous system, there were peripheral neurons. Evolutionarily speaking, brain is the inside of the skin (Swanson 2003, Ryan and Grant 2009). Functionally speaking, skin is the outside of the brain - there are only three nerve cells between any location on the skin surface of a patient and the processing area for somatosensation in a patient's brain (Mason 2011), from their skin cells to their conscious awareness, their sense of self.

If it is true that a brain is predictive, not reactive, this means that sensory input from skin, for example by a manual therapist with kind heart and words and hands, can maybe touch a patient's brain in a non-nociceptive, somatosensory processing representational area, and that little extra bit of novel input may help it make descending modulation changes in whatever prediction of "danger" it made; such new and innocuous input may help it dismantle pain production.

In the human organism,

1. the nervous system (including peripheral) takes care of business on behalf of the "whole" organism or individual, usually seamlessly but not always;
2. without conscious awareness, there is no pain
3. conscious awareness is "brain" function
4. only new, *descending* modulation, starting at the brain's most rostral areas with conscious awareness, whether provided interpersonally (by another person, verbally or non-verbally),

or in*tra*-personally (by reading, understanding, learning and adopting), can restore ordinary sensory system homeostasis.

Since we generally treat alive, awake, and conscious humans who are experiencing a pain problem, I do not think it necessary to include any other body systems in philosophical underpinnings of our new model of interactive, manually therapeutic relationship. Yes, they all are in there and they all interact, but from a *manual therapy* practitioner standpoint, realistically, can **we** affect any of the other body systems ahead of the patient's nervous system? A nervous system that evolved to be exquisitely responsive to novel stimuli, and adaptable and protective? That regulates everything essential to its own life? I doubt it. We can build a case for including **embodied prediction** into manual therapy by recognizing the nervous system only, without ever having to stray into any other body systems. In particular we may ignore, if we so choose (and I do), structural mesodermal derivative as well as any treatment models that target them. This was common in the past but does not make sense to continue doing now or in the future. Not to me, anyway, insofar as a pain problem is involved.

PHYSIOLOGICAL CONSIDERATIONS

> *"Pain: An unpleasant sensory and emotional experience associated with actual or potential tissue damage, or described in terms of such damage. Nociception: The neural process of encoding noxious stimuli."*
>
> – *International Association for the Study of Pain, online taxonomy page*

PAIN IS NOT NOCICEPTIVE EXPERIENCE

Sometime during the 20th century in the UK, a 29-year-old male construction worker jumped or fell from a height and landed on his feet on a board that had a spike sticking up from it: the spike pierced the sole of his boot and came right out the top. He exhibited behaviour indicative of severe pain. He was taken to an emergency center in considerable distress where he was given pain medication. Eventually he calmed down enough to allow staff to pull out the nail and take off his boot. As it turned out, the nail had gone between his toes, and there had been no tissue damage whatsoever (Fisher et al. 1995). This is a remarkable and rare case of pain perception and pain behaviour in the complete absence of any nociceptive input whatsoever.

NOCICEPTION IS NOT PAIN EXPERIENCE

More common than reports of devastating pain experienced without any evidence of tissue injury are reports of devastating injury that did not hurt at all at the time, for example soldiers in the heat of battle who felt a bump but did not realize they had been shot until they saw blood spread into their clothing.

On March 31, 2013, Kevin Ware, a young basketball player for the Louisville Cardinals, jumped up to redirect the ball during a game, and came down on his right leg, something he had probably done hundreds if not thousands of times before. This time his lower leg shattered into a compound fracture. Ware stayed on his back; he lifted his leg up to see why it would not let him get up: the jagged proximal ends of the completely fractured bones had cut through his shin and protruded out by several inches. His leg had a new "knee" that should not have been there. Gasps rose from the crowd and his teammates, once they realized what had happened, clutched at each other in horror. Team handlers rushed over, covered Ware's leg with a towel, and whisked him away by stretcher for medical care. Ware claimed (Nudd 2013), "I saw the bone six inches out I didn't feel any pain. It didn't hurt. Honestly, it didn't hurt. It was just scary. It was probably one of the scariest moments in my life."

A RELATIONSHIP BETWEEN NOCICEPTION AND PAIN IS NOT STRAIGHTFORWARD

"The straightforward equation between tissue damage and pain often does not hold. The chronic back pain mentioned above can seldom be traced to any discoverable tissue damage. In cases where wounding has occurred, it is common, moreover, for pain, often severe pain, to persist after the damage has healed. This is perhaps best known in the case of phantom limbs. Years after the injury has apparently healed, the patient may be subject to excruciating pain from parts of the missing limb. There are, furthermore, well-authenticated instances of acute pain persisting in a phantom limb when all (peripheral) connections to that limb have been severed. This sometimes occurs in victims of accidents in which the spine is severed. After recovery the patient has lost all sensation and movement in the body and limbs below the point of fracture. Yet in some tragic cases agonizing pain persists from these lost regions. Even after surgical procedures to remove the pain pathways (see below) in the spinal cord above the fracture plane, the cramps and burning sensations remain. These patients provide a searching test of any theory which suggests that pain is only, or even mainly, caused by messages from the site of tissue damage. Perhaps the brain sends an 'efference copy' which cannot be matched by the defective sensory return. This proposal finds support in the still controversial but nevertheless ingenious experiments with mirrors which give the patient the visual illusion that the lost region is, after all, still present. In these experiments the pain from the phantom is sometimes greatly reduced. A further searching test is provided by a far less tragic circumstance. If a local anaesthetic is injected into the brachial plexus (the rope of nerves from the arm entering the spinal cord at the level of the shoulder) the subject feels the arm to be painfully swollen and in a definite and often impos-

sible place (perhaps bent up inside the thorax) and this illusion can only occasionally be dispelled by seeing it or palpating it in the correct position. In this case it is not the tattoo of impulses arriving from the periphery but the absence of such a tattoo which 'grabs the attention' of the central nervous system (CNS).

"Vice versa, pain is frequently not felt when tissue damage is extensive. Soldiers in the heat of action often fail to notice quite severe wounds. Only later, when the battle has been lost or won and there is nothing further to do, does the pain begin. The famous instance of Dr. Livingstone and the Lion makes the same point. Dr. Livingstone recounts how in darkest Africa a lion leapt from the jungle on to his back. He recalls hearing its dreadful roar close to his ear and looking down at its jaws and powerful claws rasping his body before his rescuers freed him. But, he says, it all seemed to happen in a dream, he felt no pain, no terror. Dr. Livingstone was in no doubt that all this proved the beneficence of the Deity who would not permit the war of Nature to cause so vast a pit of pain and suffering. Evolutionists would suggest a different, though complementary, explanation. The organism 'concentrates' on one task at a time; languishing in the Lion's jaw or flinching during the clash of arms in warfare is not an adaptive behaviour: the moment of crisis is no moment for the organism to concern itself with the repair of tissue damage. There are more urgent considerations. The pain-induced quiescence required for healing can come later." ~ p. 439-40, Chapter 22, Pain, in Biology of Sensory Systems, 2nd ed., 2008, by C.U.M. Smith.

One must keep nociception and pain in separate conceptual baskets, somehow, because they do tend to blur into each other still, thanks to centuries of Cartesian ideas about pain and the power of biomedical indoctrination.

Yes, you can learn to over ride your own spinal cord's reflexive withdrawal from nociceptive input. Yes, you can train yourself to do all sorts of things in spite of having pain. Yes, you can train yourself to override your own stress responses and emotional responses to nociceptive input. That is what mindfulness training for chronic pain is all about. Two of the current best educators for this, Kevin Vowels and Bronnie Thompson, shared their gleaned wisdom with manual therapists of all kinds at the San Diego Pain Summit in 2016.

FEEDBACK LOOPS

Every physiological process in the body and in the nervous system generates its own feedback, which loops into brain systems that preserve the equilibrium of homeostasis.

In a negative feedback loop, output reduces the original effect of the stimulus. Things go back to normal. For example, in the case of stress, stress hormones released into the blood stream reach and activate *both* the cells that produce adrenalin, *and* cells in the brain that *inhibit* the pituitary cells that put out the stress hormones in the first place. Negative feedback loops are not a problem (Herman et al. 2012).

In a *positive* feedback loop, however, the output *enhances* the original stimulus. This can turn into a problem! Think of what happens with microphone squeal. As Eric Meira points out, pain will make one fearful of movement, which leads to less movement, which leads to more pain, and more fear, etc. (Meira 2014).

Some kinds of chronic pain could be regarded perhaps, as a positive feedback loop within and among different systems that did not return to normal all by itself (Chapman 2008). Prolonged sensitization of nociceptors beyond the stage where tissue healing has occurred, may involve positive feedback loops; for example, microglia and other glia in the spinal cord may operate to maintain a long-term state of facilitation in the spinal cord, of ascending nociceptive input. There are all sorts of possibilities to be explored and described, at the level of the spinal cord and above, many of which may involve stress mechanisms in a brain that was overwhelmed by too much stress all at once, or that grew up in an environment in which overwhelming stress was common and learned to think that was "normal.".

We must include the *entire* nervous system, both central and peripheral, in our clinical reasoning, for the following simple reason: the Critterbrain is in charge of regulating physiology, and the peripheral nervous system is in charge of carrying out the brain's physiological tasks. In fact the Critterbrain and attached peripheral nervous system regulate and coordinate our entire physical life (Bennaroch et al. 2008).

THE BRAIN EVOLVED TO FILTER OUT NOCICEPTIVE INFORMATION

And it usually does, easily, except for when biologically reactive, physiological positive feedback loops emerge that *amplify* nociceptive input, enhance and maintain it, or when an individual has become stressed to the point that their brain's endogenous opioid production may have become impaired or depleted, or if "neurotags" develop, then deploy in the absence of alternative input.

> Cory Blickenstaff: *"I have a question about the effects of analgesia with stress: So, some of the studies that have come out, you know when they talk about it in terms of exercise they called it exercise-induced hypoalgesia, which I'm assuming is the same thing.."*

> Robert Sapolsky: *"Yup.."*

> Cory Blickenstaff: *"... And that there have been some populations that have been identified that seem to have an impairment to be able to bring this about, and it's not.. so my question is you mentioned there are sometimes that maybe this becomes exhausted like there are populations, for example with chronic low back pain.. that this has not been shown*

to be present but there are other groups that it has like people that have diagnosed with fibromyalgia for example so I'm just curious of what your take is on that."

Robert Sapolsky: *"OK: you know, so as soon as you are wrestling with individual differences in an endocrine realm like this, the usual suspects are either individual differences in how much hormone you are making or releasing beta-endorphin, or individual differences in the number of receptors, the efficacy of them, their coupling of the target cell, sort of downstream effects... how loud are you yelling and how sensitive your ears to the signal coming through: that being a general theme throughout, at the beta-endorphin end, my guess is – I don't know this literature well – my guess is a preponderance of insufficient analgesia-type disorders, are much more at the beta-endorphin end of it rather than responding to it with receptors. This is because for some reason the pituitary doesn't have huge stores of it, and beta-endorphin is made from this precursor molecule that's like this gigantic... it's called POMC, pro-opiomelanocortin that goes through this insanely complicated processing – it takes a lot of work for the pituitary to make a lot of endorphin – it's got an Achilles heel at that end. That's why chronic stress depletes the endorphin. My bet is, most of the disorders of something with stress or exercise-induced analgesia, it's gonna be at the pituitary end rather than the target tissue end."* – transcript of Q&A excerpt from San Diego Pain Summit 2016

If nociceptive information makes it through the gate in the dorsal horn and up the spinal cord, and is so overwhelming (through temporal summation and/or spatial summation) that it may "hurt" the person inside the nervous system, then one could describe it as "painful" sensation. But it is not exactly "pain." Not yet.

If such information were to get through, perhaps as a barrage, *and* if rostral areas of the central nervous system did not manage to inhibit it normally, *and* if it became woven into pre-existing stress and patterns of neurons firing in there (referred to as "neurotags" by Lorimer Moseley; see Hargrove 2012), then it *may* (but does not yet *necessarily*) become "pain," unless such a neurotag were to become activated. If a neurotag has established itself, in the future any kind of associated sensory input might trigger a pain experience, not just nociceptive input. Moseley's presentations often include the story about a baker who lost his thumb in a machine at work. The baker had phantom thumb pain, but he only really noticed it on Saturday mornings. As it turned out, on that day the wonderful odour of fresh baked bread wafting throughout the neighbourhood and up his nose was a trigger for his phantom thumb pain. Once this connection dawned on him, he put plugs up his nose on Saturday mornings and his missing thumb stopped bothering him.

SUMMARY

Pain is output by the central nervous system, and nociception is input into it.

Anything coming into the spinal cord along a nociceptive neuron is only nociception. It is, by definition, not pain. It need not be stimulated by actual tissue damage, only potential. It therefore serves the purpose of being a danger signal, not only a damage signal.

Because of the way the vertebrate central nervous system evolved, the spinal cord, which I like to call the Fishbrain, evolved first and is therefore the oldest most conserved part of the central nervous system, along with homeostatic nuclei. It is very fast. It easily takes over in any "danger signal" emergency. If you touch a hot stove, long before the heat registers as sensory input to your conscious awareness, your spinal cord will have jerked your hand right off.

Everything that evolved later (i.e., later enlargement of the brain, both Critter and human) seems to be there to *modulate, smooth out, and/or directly inhibit* raw spinal cord activity, motor and sensory, autonomic and voluntary. The Critterbrain can do this automatically, most of the time. Sometimes it needs some help from the brain parts unique to human association, cognition and awareness.

REFERENCES

1. IASP Taxonomy page, updated from Part III: Pain Terms, A Current List with Definitions and Notes on Usage" (pp 209-214) Classification of Chronic Pain, Second Edition, IASP Task Force on Taxonomy, edited by H. Merskey and N. Bogduk, IASP Press, Seattle, ©1994. http://www.iasp-pain.org/Taxonomy#Pain, retrieved May 6 2016

2. National Research Council (US) Committee on Recognition and Alleviation of Pain in Laboratory Animals; Recognition and Alleviation of Pain in Laboratory Animals. Chapter 2: Mechanisms of Pain. The National Academies Press (US) Washington (DC) 2009

3. Melzack, R., Wall, P.D., 1965, Pain Mechanisms: A New Theory. Science, New Series. Vol 150 No 3699, Nov 19, 971-979

4. Jones, L.E., (Author), 2010, First Steps: The Early Years of IASP 1973-1984. IASP Press.

5. Foster, E., Wildner, H., Tudeau, L., Haueter, S., Ralvenius ,W.T., Jegen, M., Johannssen, H., Hösli, L., Haenraets, K., Ghanem, A., Conzelmann, K., Bösl, M., and Zeilhofer, H.U., 2015, Targeted Ablation, Silencing, and Activation Establish Glycinergic Dorsal Horn Neurons as Key Components of a Spinal Gate for Pain and Itch. *Neuron*, Mar. 85: 1289-1304

6. Engel, G.L., 1977, The need for a new medical model: A challenge for biomedicine. Science 196:129–136.

7. Quintner, J.L., Cohen, M.L., Buchanan, D., Katz, J.D., and Williamson, O.D.; Pain Medicine and Its Models: Helping or Hindering? Pain Medicine Vol 9 No 7, 2008, 824–834

8. Felton, D.L., Józefowicz, R.F., 2003, Netter's Atlas of Human Neuroscience, 1st Ed. Icon Learning Systems

9. Cupp, E, 2014, dead fish is alive 001. Video uploaded to YouTube, retrieved May 6 2016. https://www.youtube.com/watch?v=AWB3aOX_h4Y

10. Satpute, A.B., Wager, T.D., Cohen-Adad, J., Bianciardi, M., Choi, J., Buhle, J.T., Wald, L.L., and Barretta, L.F., 2013, Identification of discrete functional subregions of the human periaqueductal gray. Proc Natl Acad Sci U S A. 2013 Oct 15; 110(42): 17101–17106.

11. Standring, S., 2008, Gray's Anatomy: The Anatomical Basis of Clinical Practice, Expert Consult. Churchill Livingston 40th ed.

12. Bandler, R, and Shipley, M.T., 1994, Columnar organization in the midbrain periaqueductal gray: modules for emotional expression? TINS, Vol. 17, No. 9

13. Ossipov M.H., (Author), 2009, Pain Pathways: Descending Modulation. Squire, L.R., (Editor), Encyclopedia of Neuroscience, Elsevier Ltd

14. Ossipov, M.H., Morimura, K., Porreca, F., 2014, Descending pain modulation and chronification of pain. Curr Opin Support Palliat Care. Jun. 8(2): 143-151

15. Butler, D., 2013, The Drug Cabinet in the Brain. Video uploaded to YouTube Mar 25, retrieved May 6, 2016. https://www.youtube.com/watch?v=Gd2NaGZa7M4

16. Melzack, R., 2001, Pain and the Neuromatrix in the Brain. Journal of Dental Education vol. 65no. 12 1378-1382 Dec 1

17. Melzack, R., and Katz, J., 2013, Pain. Wiley Interdisciplinary Reviews: Cognitive Science. Jan./Feb. Vol 4, Issue 1, 1-15

18. Blickenstaff, C., 2011, Therapist as 'contextual architect'. J Man Manip Ther. Nov; 19(4): 238.

19. Vagg, M., 2015, The right words matter when talking about pain. The Conversation (US pilot)December 2 online. https://theconversation.com/the-right-words-matter-when-talking-about-pain-50450

20. ScienceWeekly, 2015, Podcast at The Guardian, March 27; The science behind our sense of touch. Ian Sample interviews David J Linden, neuroscience professor John Hopkins University School of Medicine.

21. Gawande, A., 2008, The Itch. NewYorker.com. http://www.newyorker.com/magazine/2008/06/30/the-itch

22. Moseley, L., (no date), Reconceptualising Pain According to Modern Pain Science. BodyinMind blog, retrieved May 7 2016. http://www.bodyinmind.org/resources/journal-articles/full-text-articles/reconceptualising-pain-according-to-modern-pain-science/

23. Legrain, V., Iannetti, G.D., Plaghki, L., and Mouraux, A., 2011, The pain matrix reloaded: a salience detection system for the body. Prog Neurobiol. Jan;93(1):111-24

24. BBC Two, 2010, The Rubber Hand Illusion – Horizon: Is Seeing Believing? – BBC Two. Video upload Oct 15. www.youtube.com/watch?v=sxwn1w7MJvk

25. Stanford Encyclopedia of Philosophy online, entry for phenomenology, retrieved May 7 2016-05-07 http://plato.stanford.edu/entries/phenomenology/

26. Stanford Encyclopedia of Philosophy online, entry for embod, retrieved May 7 2016-05-07 http://plato.stanford.edu/entries/embodied-cognition/

27. Maturana, H.R., and Varela, F.J., 1980. Autopoiesis and Cognition: The Realization of the Living (Boston Studies in the Philosophy of Science, Vol. 42). D. Reidel Publishing Company

28. Smith, C.U.M. (Author), 2008, Biology of Sensory Systems. Chapter 3 pp31-39, published online Nov. 24.

29. Barrett, L.F., 2016, The Predictive Brain. Available online at https://www.edge.org/annual-question/2016/response/26707 Retrieved May 11, 2016.

30. Buzsáki, G. (Author), 2006, Rhythms of the Brain. Oxford University Press, Aug 3

31. Clark, A., 2013, Whatever next? Predictive brains, situated agents, and the future of cognitive science. Behavioral and Brain Sciences. Volume 36 / Issue 03 / June, pp 181- 204

32. Swanson, L.W., (Author), 2003, Brain Architecture: Understanding the Basic Plan. Oxford University Press

33. Ryan, T.J. and Grant, S.G.N., 2009, The origin and evolution of synapses. Nat Rev Neurosci. Oct;10(10):701-12.

34. Mason, P. (Author), 2011, Medical Neurobiology. Oxford University Press, USA; 1 edition May 19

35. Fisher, J.P., Hassan, D.T., O'Connor, N., 1995, Minerva. Br Med J. 310:70

36. Nudd, T., 2013, Kevin Ware Says He Didn't Feel Any Pain Despite Horrific Injury. People (online) 04/04

37. Smith, C.U.M., 2008 (Author), Biology of Sensory Systems, 2nd Ed. Chapter 22, Pain, pp439-40, published online Nov. 24.

38. Pain Science Conference for Manual Therapists, 2016, presentations certified for continuing education. http://sandiegopainsummit.com/2016-summitlectures-only/2016-summit-wworkshops

39. Herman, J.P., McKlveen, J.M., Solomon, M.B., Carvalho-Netto, E., Myers, B., 2012, Neural regulation of the stress response: glucocorticoid feedback mechanisms. Braz J Med Biol Res. Apr., 45(4): 292–298.

40. Meira, E., 2014, Getting Rid of Something Positive. PT Podcast Network blog, April 9. Retrieved May 6 2016 http://ptpodcast.com/getting-rid-of-something-positive/

41. Chapman, C.R., Tuckett, R.P., and Song, C. W., 2008, Pain and Stress in a Systems Perspective: Reciprocal Neural, Endocrine and Immune Interactions. J Pain. Feb; 9(2): 122–145

42. Benarroch, E., Daube, J.R., Flemming, K.D., Westmoreland B.F., (Editors), 2008, Mayo Clinic Medical Neurosciences. CRC Press; 5 edition February 19

43. Sapolsky Question and Answer at San Diego Pain Summit available at http://sandiegopainsummit.com/education-videos

44. Hargrove, T., 2012, Review of Moseley/Hodges Talk Part Two. BetterMovement blog, retrieved May 7, 2016. http://www.bettermovement.org/blog/2012/review-of-moseley-hodges-talk-part-two

3. MANUAL THERAPY TREATS NERVOUS SYSTEM PAIN, NOT TISSUE

I want to take a page or so to describe my own personal bias - this seems as good a place as any.

Well into my seventh decade by now, I have personally benefited from manual therapy for various pain experiences at various times in various body zones, all of which were distressing, some more than others. Some stemmed from injury and others arose from seemingly nowhere. All required no more than a few treatments and thankfully, went away completely. The manual therapy I received was crucial for changing the adverse interoceptive experience my brain was dishing to me like a video stuck on pause, which kept me from being able to move the way I wanted to.

I was able to avoid being medicalized for any of my pain episodes, apart from checking for fracture in one instance. I was able to completely avoid pharmaceuticals. I want to make it perfectly clear that I am not anti-medical: If I were involved in an accident and sustained injury that left me unconscious and bleeding from a severed artery but still alive with multiple compound fractures that included ribs, I would definitely want swift medical intervention to keep my body alive as it healed, and good drugs to keep me comfortable. Once it was safe to wake up, and I could re-inhabit my physicality, *re-hab* it, re-enter my body and my life, hopefully I would have assistance from someone who would be willing to let me practice having locus of control again, someone sensitive to pain perception and fully up to speed on how use hands-on therapy to help me navigate through it.

With full benefit of hindsight reasoning and confirmation bias, therefore, it seems to me that judicious sensory rehabilitation, *first*, can help people with non-medical pain move easier, feel more inclined to participate in motor rehabilitation, and thereby avoid unnecessary surgery. I am all for any pain revolution that can help practitioners put people back in charge of themselves and their lives with least delay.

This manual exists because I would love to see slow interactive manual therapy become re-framed simply as sensory rehabilitation. I think it can co-exist with and possibly should even precede motor rehabilitation. In some cases, it might even replace motor rehabilitation: If pain goes away and movement feels normal again, strength, normal use of a body part, etc., often returns by itself. Why? Because weakness was likely never the problem to begin with – instead, pain was inhibiting ordinary motor control and output.

Pain might be felt as strictly physical. It might start out perceived as physical and become emotionally overlain. It may start out as a small problem that turns into something a lot bigger. It is usually a mixed bag. Sometimes it will be injury-related; however, pain that lasts far longer than it is useful, way past a time frame in which healing should be complete, is *distressing*. Often it can come seemingly out of nowhere. Intense pain that seems to have come out of nowhere is bewildering, shocking, as well as distressing. There will always be people who must deal with some pain problem, and who seek us out, because they perceive, rightly or wrongly, that the "pain" is a "thing" in their "body."

Our job is to help them, with that.

If they ask us to.

If we try to claim we can treat medical *conditions* with manual therapy, we are going to veer dangerously close to the world of quackery. Furthermore, there are many kinds of chronic pain "syndromes" for which manual therapy in and of itself is of little or no value. For example, what can manual therapy do for phantom pain? Nothing. Because, what is there, to treat, physically?

Nothing.

Mirror therapy can help though (Ramachandran and Rogers-Ramachandran 1996).

Rubber hand illusion involves persuading the brain that a fake rubber hand is part of the body for which it is responsible (BBC Two 2010). Once the illusion is established, things are done to the fake hand, like hitting it with a hammer. This elicits a response, and leaves us to ponder the mystery of the salience system in the brain that responds to a perceived threat with visual input only, with absolutely no actual tissue damage or nociceptive stimulation necessary. In a fairly recent study, Chae et al. (2015) showed that psychophysical and neurophysiological responses could be produced from acupuncture applied to a rubber hand.

Consideration of pain as being in the brain, and how linked it can be to visual perception, has opened up a great deal of new therapeutic territory. Moseley and his group have explored how various chronic pain conditions respond to visual stimulation; for example, viewing a chronically painful body part through a minimizing lens decreases pain and swelling associated with movement (Moseley, Parsons, and Spence 2008). Bodily illusions such as mirror therapy, bodily resizing, and use of functional prostheses show therapeutic promise, according to a systematic review and meta-analysis recently conducted (Boesch et al. 2016). Graded motor imagery is useful (Moseley 2004a, 2004b, 2005, 2006).

One might legitimately wonder, where does all this leave us manual therapists? I can think of a few answers... people do still have bodies that they perceive as hurting them – they will continue to hire people like us to help them, through those bodies. Second, I think manual therapy could use a great deal of reconceptualising and reframing, which is why this book has come about, and why this chapter is included.

The sort of chronic pain that *may* respond well to manual therapy is in my opinion, confined to that pain which can be of any duration, perceived as being confined to a neuroanatomically plausible region, and that can be traced to having not moved enough or having moved too much – i.e., so-called mechanical pain. It may well involve spinal cord-mediated withdrawal reflex, creating motor output that has not been sufficiently inhibited or at least modulated by rostral parts of the central nervous system. It would involve ongoing nociceptive input from within nerves, themselves. See tunnel syndromes (Lundborg 1988, and 1988, Pećina, Krmpotić-Nemanić, and Markiewitz 2001), and the IASP taxonomy page note, regarding neuritis as a special case of neuropathy reserved for inflammatory processes affecting nerves. I will discuss these later; for now, let me say only that I am quite convinced that this is the only kind of "chronic pain" that manual therapists can successfully treat with hands-on approaches regardless of what is we may *think* we are doing, or what diagnostic label the patient may have been handed, or what our favourite conception of pain might be. (Usually it is a confused mess: mechanisms, treatment approaches based on tradition, beliefs in our own efficacy of method, are all jumbled up together, with language that reflects only the mess, no real understanding, and gives us an illusion of being "operative," instead of merely interactive.)

I suspect that way back when, in pre-scientific days, especially pre-pain-science days, manual therapists simply spotted patterns of behaviour or dysfunction in patients and assigned names to them. Patterns (Shermer 2008) arise spontaneously in the mind. Visual patterns that remind people of something, for example cloud formations that look like animals shapes or faces, or the Virgin Mary on a piece of toast, are called "pareidolia." Pareidolia can also be cognitive-kinaesthetic, i.e., palpatory (Ingraham 2015). For example, many manual therapists are still convinced they can feel skull sutures and move them, or can lengthen muscle or fascia directly. When subjected to closer scrutiny, kinaesthetically pareidolic patterns are found to not exist except in the minds of those who believe in them.

Here are some common manual therapy examples of patternicity that combine the visual and kinaesthetic and lead to palpatory pareidolia, that in turn leads to unsupportable self-delusion (what I like to call "conceptual hallucination"), and/or plenty of Type I clinical errors (Bell 2015):

- Energy meridians (acupuncture)
- Subluxation (chiropractic)
- Biomechanical/postural/structural "faults," movement "dysfunctions," muscle strength or weakness (orthopaedic physiotherapy, medical physiatry, podiatry)
- Zones (reflexology)
- Muscular tension patterns, fascia restrictions, trigger points (massage, structural integration, dry needlers, "Rolfing")
- Torsions, upslips, FRSLs and ERSLs, "energy cysts" (osteopathy)

These patterns are reinforced by 'post hoc ergo propter hoc' thinking; i.e., "I did this, and that happened, therefore my reasoning is true."

Patterns like these, rightfully pointed out, are still being (wrongfully, according to me) taught as *nouns*, and practitioners still go out into the world treating these things they are trained to spot *as* nouns. They go on to believe they can treat nouns.

I would propose, instead, that these patterns be framed as motor output aberrations, often associated with pain, perhaps by a nervous system undergoing possible anxiety and/or endogenous stress, that regards itself to be under some sort of siege.

Perhaps all the siege amounts to is peripheral neural input *secondary to, and facilitated by,* some chronic withdrawal reflex generated within a spinal cord that could have used some descending modulation of some appropriate kind, long before, but for whatever reason, at the right time, it did not occur, and now it seemingly cannot (not all by itself, at least).

We could easily learn to view patterns of dysfunction as verbs, instead, as signs of defensive motor output by a nervous system, *not as defects causing pain*. We might consider the possibility that pain perception when present, or even nociceptive input under the level of our conscious radar, *precedes* motor aberrations; not that conceptualized patterns spotted in body structure or movement *cause* pain. For those who do *not* experience pain most of their life, their own movement, structure, and biomechanics do not bother them in the slightest, even though plenty of faulty "patterns" may be observed.

Harriet Hall, a medical doctor and professional sceptic, developed a perspective on evidence-gathering research that she calls "tooth fairy science." One can do a study on getting paid for baby teeth, she says; one can gather large amounts of data, measure all sorts of outcomes, e.g., if more money comes from putting the tooth under the pillow or on the windowsill, putting it in a sandwich bag or a facial tissue, what socioeconomic bracket the parents are in, etc. You can gather all sorts of data, maybe, but you will *never be able to prove the tooth fairy actually exists:* Harriet Hall (2008) and her Science Based Medicine community advocate for science-based medicine as opposed to merely evidence-based medicine. Science-based medicine is based on plausible theory, first.

The search for specific results in medical science results in only hits being counted, not misses. The conventional biomedical definition of "ineffective" is, 'no more effective than placebo'. When subjected to statistical scrutiny with confirmation bias and patternicity removed, manual therapy almost invariably washes out as being "ineffective" (Menke 2014; Kumar et al. 2013; Artus et al. 2010; Kent et al. 2005).

So also do some orthopaedic surgical procedures, though; on backs (Buchbinder et al. 2009), knees (Moseley et al. 2002), and shoulders (Ketola et al. 2013).

I think we can agree that if it comes down to something we do being no more effective than placebo, manual therapy is *at least* less invasive; it might even have marginally, but measurably, better outcomes than surgery, sometimes (Fernández-de-Las Peñas et al., 2015).

I am pretty sure we will never be able to prove that manual therapy "works," or that our favourite way of reifying it ever will achieve any "construct" or "concept" "validity."

Apparently:

1. We cannot reliably palpate spines, paraspinal soft tissue, (Seffinger et al. 2004) or so-called trigger points (Nice et al. 1992; Wolfe et al. 1992; Hsieh et al., 2000; Myburgh et al. 2008; Lucas et al. 2009) or bony landmarks (Stovall and Kumar 2010, Sutton et al. 2013)

2. We can make lots of noise but cannot accurately manipulate spines at specific levels (Ross et al. 2004; Dunning et al. 2013; Troyanovich et al. 1998; Harms et al. 1997; Snodgrass et al. 2006).

3. We cannot stretch out fascia (Threlkeld 1992; Schleip 2003; Chaudhry et al. 2008) or muscle (Weppler and Magnusson 2010; Katalinic et al. 2011)

4. Myofascial triggerpoints cannot be shown to exist, are fiction (Quintner and Cohen 1994; Wolfe 2013; Quintner et al. 2015).

5. We cannot move cranial sutures (Zegarra-Parodi et al. 2009; Downey et al. 2006).

6. Subluxations (the chiro kind) do not exist (Nansel and Szlazak 1995; Mirtz et al 2009)

7. We cannot move sacroiliac joints (Tullberg et al. 1998)

8. High velocity manipulation is not worth the bother of learning, and worrying about what segment you are mobilizing is likely futile (Chiradejnant et al. 2003; Kent et al. 2005; Aquino et al. 2009; Schomacher 2009; Artus et al. 2010)

Several have argued for a less tissue-based, less biomechanical minded, more neurophysiological approach to manual therapy; Gifford and Butler 1997; Gifford 1998; Jones, Edwards and Gifford 2002; Wellens 2010; Zusman 1994, 1998, 2002, 2011; Lederman 2010, 2011; Bialosky et al. 2009, Bialosky et al. 2011, Jacobs and Silvernail 2011.

But maybe we do not need to try to prove *anything*. Maybe *non*-specific results are perfectly *OK*. Maybe something so intimate and interactively interpersonal as non-verbal physical contact between two individuals, within otherwise verbal, therapeutic inter-subjective space and time, with a shared objective of relieving pain in the one who initiated the therapeutic contract, does not *need* specific scientific validation (Gebhard 2011; Miciak et al 2012; Medical Xpress 2013).

Maybe all we need are better, updated premises.

Pain is very common in our modern world but it does not stem from tissue findings on imaging. In one large study (Nakashima 2015), researchers examined 1211 healthy volunteers with no pain, ranging in age from 20 to 70 years, for cervical spinal disease. Most of them (87.6%) had "bad" discs, and spinal cord compression was common, *but they had no pain*. In another, Brinjikji et al. (2015) reviewed 33 articles with reports of disk degeneration, disk signal loss, disk height loss, disk bulge, disk protrusion, annular fissures, facet degeneration, and spondylolisthesis, that covered a total of 3110 *asymptomatic* adult individuals of all ages, and concluded such imaging findings were common, normal, and age-related.

"Asymptomatic" means *no pain* connected to findings. Think about that. Think about that for a long time – let it seep into your brain.

The biomedical model of pain (that pain is invariably associated with some kind of tissue damage or pathological process) cannot be relied upon, entirely - way too many Type I errors are involved (Stafford 2015).

Nowadays, the predominant model of chronic pain, i.e., pain that has persisted long past the time frame for which it is *usefully* protective, is the biopsychosocial model, or if you prefer, the socio-psycho-bio model. What a person *thinks* about their pain will greatly *affect* their pain. How significant others treat them and any disability they have with pain at home will greatly affect their pain perception (McCluskey et al. 2011).

To help them, help them *understand* how nervous systems become painful. Teach them. Give them *better* ideas for their brains to chew on. Just think – you are teaching them concepts that will likely help them in the future, instead of interfere with their lives or turn them into permanent pain patients caught in an anxiety-ridden, biological, physiological positive feedback loop.

Is it not time to reinvent manual therapy? Could we simply stop trying to study or "fix" structural or purely imaginary "things"? Could we not just reframe manual therapy as a way we can interact more with the actual patient (Øberg *et al.* 2015, Olesen 2015)?

Could we please just *stop* talking to people about conceptual hallucinations based on nothing but palpatory fantasy? They support illusory, hypothetical, bottom-up, pathoanatomical "causes" of pain, which *pain science* does not support.

Why should we stop? Well, because:

1. research cannot show if they exist in the first place (Hall 2008)
2. talking to patients about them is frankly noceboic (Atlas and Wager 2012, Louw 2014)
3. nocebo can interfere with outcomes (Bittar 2015; Benedetti et al. 2007; Colloca and Benedetti 2007).

Why would we want to interfere negatively with our own treatment outcomes by perpetrating harmful ideas to patients? Why do we just not stop perpetrating ideas *to ourselves* about pain that are simply unsupportable?

People usually come to see us *for pain*. (I.e., red flags are ruled out first.)

It's *OK* that it is all about the patients and their brains, and not about us or magic hands or treatment models and faulty conceptualizations so many are still so bound to. We do not *need* to believe a) that we have magic hands or b) that we can bend tissue to our will. We do not *need* to have patients think that improvement has anything to do with *any*thing outside of their *own* nervous system's wonderful capacity to right itself, to self-correct, with just some small additional input of an innocuous kind, from a friendly human primate social groomer, and some changed motor behaviour on their part, following.

Frankly, I feel relieved that it is not up to me to "fix" people.

I want to emphasize how important it is to put the responsibility onto the patient, and divest oneself of any responsibility other than positive encouragement, which may include careful manual therapy of a most superficial kind (a set of tricks really). By all means, touch all you want, but lighter is usually better and slower is always better, in my experience, for the patient's *nervous system* (Mancini 2014). I want to emphasize how important it is to give the patient full rein to get them*selves* better. It is complex but not impossible (Moseley 2003): tell them in advance:

1. Our current understanding about pain, how it works, why it is there: ("your wonderful nervous system is trying to protect you")

2. That they have everything they need inside their own brain already, to resolve pain, how that works: ("Your brain has a lot of little nuclei that can make any kind of drug it needs - all we have to do is stimulate it the right way")

3. How the brain is a big learning machine, and how they can trust their magnificent brain to do what it needs to do by simply stepping out of its way

4. that the work you intend to do with them physically is to help them feel better on the inside of themselves, and help them move better after.

REFERENCES

1. Ramachandran, V.S., Rogers-Ramachandran, D., 1996, Synesthesia in phantom limbs induced with mirrors. Proc Biol Sci, Apr 22; 263(1369):377-86

2. BBC Two, 2010, The Rubber Hand Illusion – Horizon: Is Seeing Believing? – BBC Two. Video upload Oct 15. www.youtube.com/watch?v=sxwn1w7MJvk

3. Chae, Y., Lee, I.S., Jung, W.M., Park, K., Park, H.J., Wallraven, C., 2015, Psychophysical and neurophysiological responses to acupuncture stimulation to incorporated rubber hand. Neurosci Lett. Mar 30;591:48-52

4. Moseley, G.L., Parsons, T.J., Spence, C., 2008, Visual distortion of a limb modulates the pain and swelling evoked by movement. Current Biology, Nov 25, Vol 18 Issue 22. pR1047-R1048

5. Boesch, E., Bellan, V., Moseley, G.L., Stanton, T.R., 2016, The effect of bodily illusions on clinical pain: a systematic review and meta-analysis. PAIN, Vol 157(3), March, p 516-529

6. Moseley, G. L., 2004a, Graded motor imagery is effective for long standing complex regional pain syndrome. Pain, 108, 192-198.

7. Moseley, G. L., 2004b, Why do people with complex regional pain syndrome take longer to recognise their affected hand? Neurology, 62, 2182-2186.

8. Moseley, G. L., 2005, Is successful rehabilitation of complex regional pain syndrome due to sustained attention to the affected limb. Pain, 114, 54-61.

9. Moseley, G. L., 2006, Graded motor imagery for pathologic pain. Neurology, 67, 1-6.

10. Lundborg, G., 1988, Intraneural microcirculation. Orthop Clin North Am. Jan;19(1):1-12.

11. Lundborg, G., (Author), 1988, Nerve Injury and Repair. New York. Churchill Livingstone

12. Pećina, M.M., Krmpotić-Nemanić, J., Markiewitz, A.D., (Authors), 2001, Tunnel Syndromes. CRC Press; 3 edition, August 16

13. Note regarding "Neuritis", IASP taxonomy page, http://www.iasp-pain.org/Taxonomy#Peripheralneuropathicpain

14. Shermer, M., 2008, Patternicity: Finding Meaningful Patterns in Meaningless Noise. Scientific American Dec 1, retrieved May 8 2016. http://www.scientificamerican.com/article/patternicity-finding-meaningful-patterns/

15. Ingraham, P., 2015, Palpatory Pareidolia. PainScience.com Sept 17. Retrieved May 8, 2016. www.painscience.com/articles/palpatory-pareidolia.php

16. Bell, V., 2015, Mind Hacks blog; No more Type I/II error confusion. Nov 16 Retrieved May 10, 2016. https://mindhacks.com/2015/11/16/no-more-type-iii-error-confusion/

17. Hall, H., 2008, Another acupuncture study – on heartburn. Science-Based Medicine blog, Feb 12, retrieved May 8, 2016. www.sciencebasedmedicine.org/another-acupuncture-study-on-heartburn/

18. Menke, J.M., 2014, Do manual therapies help low back pain? A comparative effectiveness meta-analysis. Spine (Phila Pa 1976). Apr 1;39(7):E463-72.

19. Kumar, S., Beaton, K., and Hughes, T., 2013, The effectiveness of massage therapy for the treatment of nonspecific low back pain: a systematic review of systematic reviews. Int J Gen Med.; 6: 733–741

20. Artus, M., van der Windt, D.A., Jordan, K.P., Hay, E.M., 2010, Low back pain symptoms show a similar pattern of improvement following a wide range of primary care treatments: a systematic review of randomized clinical trials. Rheumatology (Oxford). Dec;49(12):2346-56.

21. Kent, P., Marks, D., Pearson, W., Keating, J., 2005, Does clinician treatment choice improve the outcomes of manual therapy for nonspecific low back pain? A metaanalysis. J Manipulative Physiol Ther. Jun;28(5):312-22.

22. Buchbinder, R., Osborne, R.H., Ebeling, P.R., Wark, J.D., Mitchell, P., Wriedt, C., Graves, S., Staples, M.P., Murphy, B., 2009, A randomized trial of vertebroplasty for painful osteoporotic vertebral fractures. N Engl J Med. Aug 6;361(6):557-68

23. Moseley, J.B., O'Malley, K., Petersen, N.J., Menke, T.J., Brody, B.A., Kuykendall, D.H., John C. Hollingsworth, J.C., Ashton, C.M., and Wray N.P., 2002, A Controlled Trial of Arthroscopic Surgery for Osteoarthritis of the Knee. N Engl J Med 2002; 347:81-88 July 11

24. Ketola, S., Lehtinen, J., Rousi, T., Nissinen, M., Huhtala, H., Konttinen, Y.T., and Arnala, I., 2013, No evidence of long-term benefits of arthroscopic acromioplasty in the treatment of shoulder impingment syndrome. Five-year results of a randomized controlled trial. Bone Joint Res. Jul; 2(7): 132–139

25. Fernández-de-Las Peñas, C., Ortega-Santiago, R., de la Llave-Rincón, A.I., Martínez-Perez, A., Fahandezh-Saddi Díaz, H., Martínez-Martín, J., Pareja JA,Cuadrado-Pérez, M.L., 2015, Manual Physical Therapy Versus Surgery for Carpal Tunnel Syndrome: A Randomized Parallel-Group Trial. J Pain. Nov;16(11):1087-94

26. Seffinger, M.A., Najm, W.I., Mishra, S.I., Adams, A., Dickerson, V.M., Murphy, L.S., Reinsch, S., 2004, Reliability of spinal palpation for diagnosis of back and neck pain: a systematic review of the literature. Spine (Phila Pa 1976). Oct 1;29(19):E413-25.

27. Nice, D.A., Riddle, D.L., Lamb, R.L., Mayhew, T.P., Rucker, K., 1992, Intertester reliability of judgments of the presence of trigger points in patients with low back pain. Arch Phys Med Rehabil. Oct;73(10):893-8.

28. Wolfe, F., Simons, D.G., Fricton, J., Bennett, R.M., Goldenberg, D.L., Gerwin, R., Hathaway, D., McCain, G.A., Russell, I.J., Sanders, H.O., et al., 1992, The fibromyalgia and myofascial pain syndromes: a preliminary study of tender points and trigger points in persons with fibromyalgia, myofascial pain syndrome and no disease. J Rheumatol. Jun;19(6):944-51.

29. Hsieh, C.Y., Hong, C.Z., Adams, A.H., Platt, K.J., Danielson, C.D., Hoehler, F.K., Tobis, J.S., 2000, Interexaminer reliability of the palpation of trigger points in the trunk and lower limb muscles. Arch Phys Med Rehabil. Mar;81(3):258-64.

30. Myburgh, C., Larsen, A.H., Hartvigsen, J., 2008, A systematic, critical review of manual palpation for identifying myofascial trigger points: evidence and clinical significance. Arch Phys Med Rehabil. Jun; 89(6):1169-76

31. Lucas, N., Macaskill, P., Irwig, L., Moran, R., Bogduk, N., 2009, Reliability of physical examination for diagnosis of myofascial trigger points: a systematic review of the literature. Clinical Journal of Pain; 25(1): 80-89.

32. Stovall, B.A., and Kumar, S., 2010, Reliability of Bony Anatomic Landmark Asymmetry Assessment in the Lumbopelvic Region: Application to Osteopathic Medical Education. J Am Osteopath Assoc. November ; 110(11): 667–674.

33. Sutton, C., Nono, L., Johnston, R.G., and Thomson, O.P., 2013, The effects of experience on the inter-reliability of osteopaths to detect changes in posterior superior iliac spine levels using a hidden heel wedge. J Bodyw Mov Ther. Apr;17(2):143-50

34. Ross, J.K., Bereznick, D.E., and McGill, S.M., 2004, Determining cavitation location during lumbar and thoracic spinal manipulation: is spinal manipulation accurate and specific? Spine (Phila Pa 1976). Jul 1;29(13):1452-7

35. Dunning, J., Mourad F., Barbero M., Leoni, D., Cescon, C., and Butts, R., 2013, Bilateral and multiple cavitation sounds during upper cervical thrust manipulation. BMC Musculoskeletal Disorders 14:24

36. Troyanovich, S.J., Harrison, D.D., and Harrison, D.E., 1998, Motion palpation: it's time to accept the evidence.J.Manipulative Physiol Ther. 21:568–571.

37. Harms, M.C., and Bader, DL., 1997, Variability of forces applied by experienced therapists during spinal mobilization. Clin Biomech (Bristol, Avon). Sep;12(6):393-399.

38. Snodgrass, S.J., Rivett, D.A., and Robertson, V.J., 2006, Manual forces applied during posterior-to-anterior spinal mobilization: a review of the evidence. J Manipulative Physiol Ther. May;29(4):316-29.

39. Threlkeld, A.J., 1992, The Effects of Manual Therapy on Connective Tissue. Physical Therapy Dec. vol. 72 no. 12 893-902

40. Schleip, R., 2003, Fascial plasticity - a new neurobiological explanation: Part 1. Journal of Bodywork and Movement Therapies Volume 7, Issue 1, Jan. Pages 11–19

41. Chaudhry, H., Schleip, R., Ji, Z., Bukiet, B., Maney, M., and Findley, T., 2008, Three-dimensional mathematical model for deformation of human fasciae in manual therapy. J Am Osteopath Assoc. Aug;108(8):379-90

42. Weppler, C.H. and Magnusson, S.P., 2010, Increasing Muscle Extensibility: A Matter of Increasing Length or Modifying Sensation? Physical Therapy. March vol. 90 no. 3 438-449

43. Katalinic, O.M., Harvey, L.A., and Herbert, R.D., 2011, Effectiveness of Stretch for the Treatment and Prevention of Contractures in People With Neurological Conditions: A Systematic Review. Physical Therapy Jan. vol. 91 no. 1 11-24

44. Quintner, J.L., and Cohen, M.L., 1994, Referred pain of peripheral nerve origin: an alternative to the "myofascial pain" construct. Clin J Pain. Sep;10(3):243-51.

45. Wolfe, F., 2013, Travell, Simons and Cargo Cult Science. The Fibromyalgia Perplex blog, Feb 14. http://www.fmperplex.com/2013/02/14/travell-simons-and-cargo-cult-science/ Retrieved May 12, 2016

46. Quintner JL, Bove GM, and Cohen ML. A critical evaluation of the trigger point phenomenon. Rheumatology (Oxford). 2015 Mar;54(3):392-9.

47. Zegarra-Parodi, R., de Chauvigny de Blot, P., Rickards, L.D., and Renard, E.O., 2009, Cranial palpation pressures used by osteopathy students: effects of standardized protocol training. J Am Osteopath Assoc. Feb;109(2):79-85.

48. Downey, P.A., Barbano, T., Kapur-Wadhwa, R., Sciote, J.J., Siegel, M.I., and Mooney M.P., 2006, Craniosacral therapy: the effects of cranial manipulation on intracranial pressure and cranial bone movement. J Orthop Sports Phys Ther. Nov;36(11):845-53.

49. Nansel, D., and Szlazak, M., 1995, Somatic dysfunction and the phenomenon of visceral disease simulation: a probable explanation for the apparent effectiveness of somatic therapy in patients presumed to be suffering from true visceral disease. J Manipulative Physiol Ther. 18:379-397

50. Mirtz, T.A., Morgan, L., Wyatt, L.H., and Greene, L., 2009, An epidemiological examination of the subluxation construct using Hill's criteria of causation. *Chiropractic & Osteopathy* 2009, 17:13

51. Tullberg, T., Blomberg, S., Branth, B., and Johnsson, R., 1998, Manipulation does not alter the position of the sacroiliac joint. A roentgen stereophotogrammetric analysis. Spine. 23:1124–1128.

52. Chiradejnant, A., Maher, C.G., Latimer, J., and Stepkovitch, N., 2003, Efficacy of "therapist-selected" versus "randomly selected" mobilisation techniques for the treatment of low back pain: A randomised controlled trial. Australian Journal of Physiotherapy Volume 49, Issue 4, p. 233–241

53. Kent, P., Marks, D., Pearson, W., and Keating, J., 2005, Does clinician treatment choice improve the outcomes of manual therapy for nonspecific low back pain? A metaanalysis. J Manipulative Physiol Ther. Jun;28(5):312-22.

54. Aquino, R.L., Caires, P.M., Furtado, F.C., Loureiro, A.V., Ferreira, P.H., and Ferreira, M.L., 2009, Applying Joint Mobilization at Different Cervical Vertebral Levels does not Influence Immediate Pain Reduction in Patients with Chronic Neck Pain: A Randomized Clinical Trial. J Manual & Manipulative Therapy. Volume 17 Issue 2, 01 April p. 95-100

55. Schomacher, J., 2009, The Effect of an Analgesic Mobilization Technique When Applied at Symptomatic or Asymptomatic Levels of the Cervical Spine in Subjects with Neck Pain: A Randomized Controlled Trial. J Manual & Manipulative Therapy Volume 17 Issue 2, 01 April pp. 101-108

56. Artus, M., van der Windt, D.A., Jordan, K.P., Hay, E.M., 2010, Low back pain symptoms show a similar pattern of improvement following a wide range of primary care treatments: a systematic review of randomized clinical trials. Rheumatology (Oxford). Dec;49(12):2346-56

57. Gifford, L.S., and Butler, D.S.; 1997, The integration of pain sciences into clinical practice. J. Hand Therapy. Apr-Jun; 10(2): 86-95

58. Gifford, L., 1998, Pain, the Tissues and the Nervous System: A conceptual model. Physiotherapy Jan Vol 84 Issue 1 Pages 27-36.

59. Jones, M., Edwards, I., and Gifford, L., 2002, Conceptual models for implementing biopsychosocial theory in clinical practice. Man Ther. Feb;7(1):2-9. Review.

60. Wellens, F., 2010, The traditional mechanistic paradigm in the teaching and practice of manual therapy : Time for a reality check. www.physioaxis.ca

61. Zusman, M., 1994, The meaning of mechanically induced responses. Australian Journal of Physiotherapy Volume 40, Issue 1, p. 35–39

62. Zusman, M., Structure-oriented beliefs and disability due to back pain. Aust J Physiother. 1998;44(1):13-20.

63. Zusman M., 2002, Forebrain-mediated sensitization of central pain pathways: 'non-specific' pain and a new image for MT. Man Ther. May;7(2):80-8.

64. Zusman, M., 2011, The Modernization of Manipulative Therapy. International Journal of Clinical Medicine 2, 644-649

65. Lederman, E., 2010, The myth of core stability. J Bodyw Mov Ther. Jan;14(1):84-98

66. Lederman, E., 2011, The fall of the postural-structural-biomechanical model in manual and physical therapies: exemplified by lower back pain. J Bodyw Mov Ther. Apr;15(2):131-8.

67. Bialosky, J.E., Bishop, M.D., Price, D.D., Robinson, M.E., and George, S.Z., 2009, The mechanisms of manual therapy in the treatment of musculoskeletal pain: a comprehensive model. Man Ther. Oct;14(5):531-8

68. Bialosky, J.E., Bishop, M.D., George, S.Z., and Robinson, M.E., 2011, Placebo response to manual therapy: something out of nothing? J Man Manip Ther. Feb; 19(1): 11–19.

69. Jacobs, D.F., and Silvernail, J.L., 2011, Therapist as operator or interactor? Moving beyond the technique. J Man Manip Ther. May; 19(2): 120–121.

70. Gebhard, B., (no date), Relevance of Common Factors in Physical Therapy: A qualitative Analysis. (poster pdf) Retrieved May 8, 2016. www.uni-oldenburg.de/fileadmin/user_upload/sonderpaedagogik/download/Gebhard/Poster_Gebhard_common_factors_physiotherapy.pdf

71. Miciak, M., Gross, D.P., Joyce, A., 2012, A review of the psychotherapeutic 'common factors' model and its application in physical therapy: the need to consider general effects in physical therapy practice. Scand J Caring Sci. Jun;26(2):394-403.

72. (No author listed), 2013, Physiotherapy patient interaction a key ingredient to pain reduction, research says. June 5, Medical Xpress. Retrieved May 8, 2016. http://medicalxpress.com/news/2013-06-physiotherapy-patient-interaction-key-ingredient.html

73. Nakashima, H., Yukawa, Y., Suda, K., Yamagata, M., Ueta, T., and Kato, F., 2015, Abnormal Findings on Magnetic Resonance Images of the Cervical Spines in 1211 Asymptomatic Subjects. SPINE Volume 40, Number 6, pp 392-398

74. Brinjikji, W., Luetmer, P.H., Comstock, B., Bresnahan, B.W., Chen, L.E., Deyo, R.A., Halabi, S., Turner, J.A., Avins, A.L., James, K., Wald, J.T., Kallmes, D.F., and Jarvik, J.G., 2015, Systematic Literature Review of Imaging Features of Spinal Degeneration in Asymptomatic Populations. Am J Neuroradiol, April; 36(4): 811-816

75. Stafford, T., 2015, No more Type I/II error confusion. Mindhacks blogpost retrieved May 15, 2016. https://mindhacks.com/2015/11/16/no-more-type-iii-error-confusion/

76. McCluskey, S., Brooks, J., King, N., and Burton, K., 2011, The influence of 'significant others' on persistent back pain and work participation: A qualitative exploration of illness perceptions. BMC Musculoskelet Disord. 12: 236.

77. Øberg, G.K., Normann, B., and Gallagher, S., 2015, Embodied-enactive clinical reasoning in physical therapy. Physiotherapy Theory and Practice, online Jan 14

78. Olesen, J., (Not yet published as of May 8, 2016) Physical therapy and Løgstrup's ethics of proximity.

79. Atlas, L.Y., and Wager, T.D., 2012, How expectations shape pain. Neurosci. Lett.

80. Louw, A., 2014, Therapeutic Neuroscience Education: Teaching People About Pain. Blogpost at ICP Institute for Chronic Pain, May 30 (instituteforchronicpain.org)

81. Bittar, C., and Nascimento, O.J.M., 2015, Placebo and nocebo effects in the neurological practice. Arq. Neuro-Psiquiatr. vol.73 no.1 São Paulo Jan.

82. Benedetti, F., Lanotte, M., Lopiano, L., and Colloca, L., 2007, When words are painful: Unraveling the mechanisms of the nocebo effect. Neuroscience 147 p.260 –271

83. Colloca, L., and Benedetti, F., 2007, Nocebo hyperalgesia: how anxiety is turned into pain. Curr Opin Anaesthesiol. Oct; 20(5):435-9.

84. Mancini, F., Nash, T., Iannetti, G.D., and Haggard, P., 2014, Pain relief by touch: A quantitative approach. PAIN Volume 155, Issue 3 , Pages 635-642, March

85. Moseley, G.L., 2003, A pain neuromatrix approach to patients with chronic pain. Man Ther. Aug. 8(3):130-40

4. WE CANNOT ACTUALLY "TOUCH" ANYTHING EXCEPT SKIN

This seems obvious, but way too many manual therapy treatment systems *still* try to target bones or muscle lying deep beneath the *surface* layer, a thick rubbery mobile layer of highly innervated, physiologically important, force-dissipating, slidey, frictionless skin organ, and ignoring said skin organ and all the nerves in it, in the process.

The receptive fields of many kinds of sensory neurons form overlapped receptive fields at the surface: just touching skin in a properly prepared patient will send a cascade of novel sensory information through to the brain and to all its maps, to help said brain repair them. We need to respect the skin organ, think about it, and learn how to work with it, instead of against it.

Skin is, in many ways, the outside of the brain (Walsh et al. 2011; Ryan and Grant 2009; Gazzola et al. 2012; Tobin 2006; Boulais and Misery 2008; Björnsdotter et al. 2009; Hansson et al. 2009; Collins et al. 2005; Chung YG et al. 2014; Edin 1995; Vidyasagar et al. 2014). The brain has evolved from neurons that originally were membrane sensory pores (Swanson 2003). So you might say, the brain is the inside of the skin. The skin organ is held up and on and against the body by thousands of skin ligaments connecting dermis to the deep fascia, forming a final outer physiologically and neurologically sensitive layer fastened to the containment system of body wall (Wong *et al.* 2016, Nash *et al.* 2004). It exists to help the organism with protection, communication and thermoregulation. (Cutaneous nerves disseminate multiple rami to the surface of the body via skin ligaments that are tubular, discussed in a later chapter.)

The surface layer of skin, epidermis, arises from ectoderm, while neuronal structure supplying it arises from neural crest cells, also from ectoderm. The skin organ, comprised of epidermis, dermis and hypodermis, weighs as much as the skeleton (Body Worlds Exhibit 2007) and accounts for about 8% of body mass (Standring 2008) – in the obese, probably way more.

1. Skin **protects**, its heavy innervation alerting the brain of anything sharp or dangerous poking into it from the environment, providing a certain amount of friction reduction between organism and surfaces, and padding the organism against gravity.

2. Thanks to a bidirectional peripheral nervous system, skin **communicates**, turning dark if we are embarrassed or angry, and pale if we are frightened or queasy.

3. Most importantly of all, skin **thermoregulates**: the skin organ contains 10 times more blood than it requires for its own metabolism, and its vascular volume capacity can increase or decrease by as much as 20 times in case of an emergency (Standring 2008). Faced by a sudden environmental threat, the sympathetic nervous system can instantly shunt massive amounts of blood from your skin organ (and also from viscera) into your muscles, pumping them up so that you can become suddenly strong (e.g., lift a car off your child) or run very fast. All that blood circulating around in the skin organ provides radiative cooling for a big busy human brain (is it any wonder evolution selected for us to be relatively hairless?).

Much of the neural array in the skin organ is sympathetic motor, there to contract or relax smooth muscle regulating lumen size of blood vessels (Charkoudian 2003, 2010), smooth muscle in skin, to create shivering, and sweat glands to provide cooling. Blood vessels in skin are arranged in at least six complex layered plexuses of various sizes (Standring 2008), each size sensitive to specific neuropeptides secreted by both autonomic motor and C-fibre afferent neurons, which together manage microcirculation circuitry at the surface (Holzer 1997).

This complexity permits fine local control over and adaptation to various local conditions. For example, where your backside rests against a chair, the skin may build up quite a lot of warmth while the rest of your exposed skin surface is cooler. Most of the time we are completely oblivious to our own nervous system's thermoregulatory system and how hard it works to take care of us, reflexively, by keeping us and our physiology at optimal temperature relative to our environment, which may be uneven from place to place within its approximately two square meter skin organ area (Joyner 2009). It is probably a good idea to expose one's skin organ's autonomic motor output system to varied temperatures, and thereby exercise it, not let it adapt to constant warm temperature in one place (e.g., skin on backside and low back warm against a chair) with the rest exposed to ambient temperature.

Numerous afferent C-fibres and larger, faster thickly myelinated A-beta fibres convey a symphony of complex *exteroceptive* temperature and mechanoreception to the spinal cord, that falls into the innocuous or even pleasant category.

We should try to have our hands be of a temperature that the patient finds soothing, not disturbing.

Affective touch

Affective touch means, in a manual therapy context, sensory input that motivates some form of action, through non-myelinated, interoceptive, C-fibre neurons. Affective signalling spreads throughout many regions of the brain (Gordon et al. 2011). I want to stress that it is *not necessary to hurt* people in order to treat them manually.

If manual treatment is uncomfortable for any reason, nociceptive C-fibres will activate, the spinal cord will register the resulting nociceptive input first, and a withdrawal reflex will activate. Muscles will tighten and a sympathetic nervous system response may occur. Brain regions connected to processing of nociceptive input will register threat. The person in the brain might be more than willing to put up with discomfort if they believe it will help, but the subcortical and old cortical areas such as the anterior cingulate cortex and insular cortex (Critterbrain) may activate anyway, and not in a way that is favourable in the long term, probably. Do we really think setting brain parts against each other, or maintaining a standoff they may already be involved in, is a good way to proceed?

Yes-ciception

Pleasant or at least, not noxious, i.e., *innocuous* input, can result in a much different output. A subset of C fibres in skin known as C-tactile fibres, convey only *pleasurable* touch (Björnsdotter M et al 2009, Olausson et al 2002; Löken 2009). Jason Erickson, a massage therapist in Minnesota, coined the clever term, *"yes-ciceptive"* (personal communication 2012), to denote input from these kinds of neurons in the context of manual therapy contact. Innocuous touch-coding C fibre afferents synapse in the dorsal horn and reach the brain via the spinothalamic tract just as nociceptive afferent fibres do (Felton 2003). C-tactile fibres project to the insular cortex of the brain (Olausson et al. 2002).

What sort of "action" do we want to elicit?

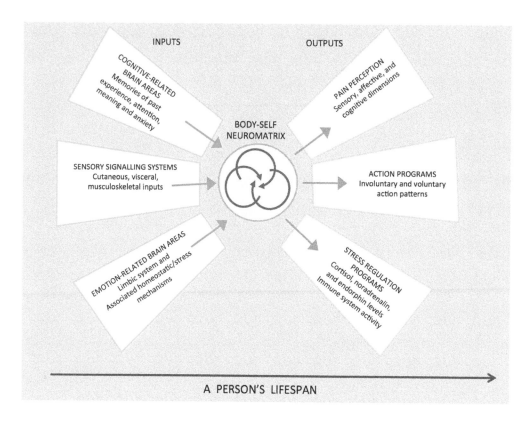

Image adapted from Melzack's neuromatrix (2001). Action is central nervous system output, along with pain and stress regulation.

Action, as we can see in the diagram above, is efferent CNS output that may express as voluntary or involuntary physical movement, volitional or non-volitional. Motor output to the body may be via cortico-spinal tracts affecting striate muscle; it may be autonomic activity via subcortical-spino pathways, regulating physiology such as blood flow. I would place descending modulation by the brain of dorsal horn synapses into the "action" category.

Brain activity may also include initiating stress regulation, which, via descending modulation, may result in decreased muscular tension: i.e., inhibition of spinal cord mediated muscular lower motor neuron output and decreased *smooth* muscle cell tension, via inhibition of spinal cord mediated sympathetic outflow. The role of cerebellum in descending modulation is gradually becoming better understood (Saab et al. 2003, Moulton et al. 2010, Hagains et al. 2011, Strata 2015). The context-dependent role played by other subcortical structures (e.g., locus ceruleus, periaqueductal grey, raphe nuclei) in descending modulation are better understood.

Other exteroceptive input

Large myelinated sensory fibres attached to type II slow-adapting stretch receptors in skin may help the brain decode tactile directional discrimination, give it somatic puzzles to solve, assisting it to focus attention away from pain and onto problem solving (Lundblad et al. 2010). Innocuous skin-stretch information travels as, and with proprioceptive information all the way up dorsal column pathways without stopping. These large neurons give off collaterals to the dorsal horn, but have no synapses until they reach dorsal column nuclei in the medulla of the brain. They can contribute to movement illusion and improved proprioception (Edin and Johansson 1995, Collins *et al.* 2005, Proske and Gandevia 2009, Lundblad *et al.* 2010, Panek *et al.* 2014). The collaterals they give off to the dorsal horn synapse with interneurons. Recently it has been shown that inhibitory interneurons within the spinal cord, stimulated by innocuous sensory input via large myelinated fibres, can inhibit nociceptive input (Foster E. et al. 2015). This provides long-awaited direct evidence to support the gate control theory of pain, first described by Melzack and Wall in 1965 (Melzack & Wall 1965). Furthermore, it seems that over time, large fibre input into the spinal cord promotes neurogenesis of inhibitory interneurons (Shechter et al. 2011). The Foster et al. and Shechter et al. papers provide support for large fiber input as being interruptive for nociception, which rules manual therapy in as plausible for treating pain perception from a bottom-up perspective, not only from a top-down perspective.

A small group of papers supports the idea that opioids are produced peripherally and may be taken up by peripheral afferent neurons (Kapitzke et al. 2005, Stein et al. 2003, 2011, 2013).

Innocuous sensory information travels about in the brain, is encoded and processed, compared to previous experiences, and evaluated for threat by the salience network (Legrain 2011). What we hope, as manual therapists, is that the brain will decide, based on innocuous and "yes-ceptive", comforting, meaning-laden somatosensory input, combined with prior and ongoing favourable cognitive and sensory input from a favourable context, that there is no threat against which it must try to defend its organism; that it will relax its guard and instead, exploit the opportunity to improve descending modulation (Ossipov 2009).

Long descending neurons from nuclei within the brainstem portion of the internal regulation system reach all the way down to the first synapse in the dorsal horn, where first-order nociceptive neurons from the periphery are trying to pass their information to second-order ascending nociceptive neurons; these descending neurons secrete substances which will either directly inhibit or facilitate such activity. Sometimes, biological activity contributes ongoingly to help maintain pain situations (Chapman 2008), and outlives its original usefulness. The internal regulation system can become more active or less active in suppressing nociceptive input depending on stress levels, environmental context, internal rumination, and past experience. If we can entice the brain to new action by giving it novel stimuli in a new context, we hope it will change its descending modulatory output to something more favourable for the person for whom lack of appropriate modulation has become persistent and detrimental, inhibiting their ability to move themselves or a part of themselves.

It is common to feel "movement" occur within the body as we treat, fleeting phenomena such as thermal change, sweating, or a feeling of fluid bubbling within or just below skin. This is perfectly normal, and is probably secondary to descending modulation operating on striate and smooth muscle output at an internal regulatory spinal cord level. After a few moments, one can usually feel softening. Softening is our main palpatory clue that the nervous system is dismantling its guardedness, a desirable effect. Other characteristics of a nervous system's self-correction are warming, and spontaneous, effortless movement (Dorko 2003, Dorko (no date), Rickards (no date), McCarthy et al. 2007).

SUMMARY

Skin is the only part of the body we can actually touch and affect easily. We can readily provide non-noxious input through non-nociceptive, thickly myelinated sensory fibres attached to endings in the skin organ that are Type II slow-adapting, e.g., Ruffini endings which respond to lateral stretch of the skin. Such input can result in

1. movement illusion and improved proprioception (Edin and Johansson 1995, Collins *et al.* 2005, Proske and Gandevia 2009, Lundblad *et al.* 2010, Panek *et al.* 2014)
2. inhibition of nociception at the spinal cord level (Foster E. et al. 2015) and fostering of neurogenesis of more inhibitory interneurons there (Shechter et al. 2011)
3. possibly, opioid uptake by peripheral sensory neurons (Kapitzke et al. 2005, Stein et al. 2003, 2011, 2013).

REFERENCES

1. Walsh, L.D., Moseley, G.L., Taylor, J.L., Gandevia, S.C., 2011, Proprioceptive signals contribute to the sense of body ownership. J Physiol. June 15, 589(Pt 12): 3009–3021.

2. Ryan, T.J., and Seth G. N. Grant, S.G.N., 2009, The origin and evolution of synapses. Nat Rev Neurosci. Oct., 10(10):701-12. Epub Sep 9.

3. Gazzola, V., Spezio, M.L., Etzel, J.A., Castelli, F., Adolphs, R., and Keysers, C., 2012, Primary somatosensory cortex discriminates affective significance in social touch. PNAS. Vol. 109 no. 25, E1657–E1666

4. Tobin, D.J., 2006, Biochemistry of human skin—our brain on the outside. Chem Soc Rev. Jan, 35(1):52-67.

5. Boulais, N., Misery, L., 2008, The epidermis: a sensory tissue. European Journal of Dermatology. Volume 18, Number 2, 119-27, march-april

6. Björnsdotter, M., Löken, L., Olausson, H., Vallbo, A., Wessberg, J., 2009, Somatotopic organization of gentle touch processing in the posterior insular cortex. J Neurosci. Jul., 22;29(29):9314-20.

7. Hansson, T., Nyman, T., Björkman, A., Lundberg, P., Nylander, L., Rosén, B., Lundborg, G., 2009, Sights of touching activates the somatosensory cortex in humans. Scand J Plast Reconstr Surg Hand Surg. 43(5):267-9.

8. Collins, D.F, Refshauge, K.M., Todd, G., Gandevia, S.C., 2005, Cutaneous receptors contribute to kinesthesia at the index finger, elbow, and knee. J Neurophysiol. Sept., 94(3):1699-706

9. Chung, Y.G., Han, S.W., Kim, H.S., Chung, S.C., Park, J.Y., Wallraven, C., Kim, S.P., 2014, Intra- and inter-hemispheric effective connectivity in the human somatosensory cortex during pressure stimulation. BMC Neuroscience, 15:43

10. Lundblad, L.C., Olausson, H.W., Malmeström, C., Wasling, H.B., 2010, Processing in prefrontal cortex underlies tactile direction discrimination: An fMRI study of a patient with a traumatic spinal cord lesion. Neurosci Lett. Oct 15;483(3):197-200.

11. Edin, B.B., and Johansson, N., 1995, Skin strain patterns provide kinaesthetic information to the human central nervous system. J Physiology. 487.1 243-251

12. Vidyasagar, R., Folger, S.E., and Parkes, L.M., 2014, Re-wiring the brain: Increased functional connectivity within primary somatosensory cortex following synchronous co-activation. Neuroimage. May 15, 92(100): 19–26.

13. Swanson, L.W., (Author), 2003, Brain Architecture: Understanding the Basic Plan. Oxford University Press

14. Wong, R., Geyer, S., Weninger, W., Guimberteau, J-C., and Jason K. Wong J.K., 2016, The dynamic anatomy and patterning of skin. Experimental Dermatology Volume 25, Issue 2, pages 92–98, Feb.

15. Nash, L.G., Phillips, M.N., Nicholson, H., Barnett, R., and Zhang, M., 2004, Skin Ligaments: Regional distribution and morphology. Clinical Anatomy, Vol 17 Issue 4 p 287-293

16. BodyWorlds Exhibit 2007, Science World, Vancouver, B.C.

17. Standring, S., 2008, Gray's Anatomy: The Anatomical Basis of Clinical Practice, Expert Consult. Churchill Livingston 40th ed.

18. Charkoudian, N., 2003, Skin Blood Flow in Adult Human Thermoregulation: How It Works, When It Does Not, and Why. Mayo Clinic Proceedings. Volume 78, Issue 5 , Pages 603-612, May

19. Charkoudian, N., 2010, Mechanisms and modifiers of reflex induced cutaneous vasodilation and vasoconstriction in humans. J Appl Physiol (1985). Oct; 109(4): 1221–1228.

20. Holzer, P., (Author), 1997, Control of the Cutaneous Vascular System by Afferent Neurons. Ch.7 in Autonomic Innervation of the Skin. (Morris, J.L., Gibbins, I.L., and Burnstock, G., editors). Overseas Publishers Association. pp 213-249

21. Joyner, M.J., 2009, Cutaneous blood flow: uncomfortable in our own skin? American Journal of Physiology - Heart and Circulatory Physiology 1 Jan. Vol. 296 no. H29-H30

22. Gordon, I., Voos, A.C., Bennett, R.H., Bolling, D.Z., Pelphrey, K.A., and Kaiser, M.D., 2011, Brain mechanisms for processing affective touch. Hum Brain Mapp. Nov 29.

23. Björnsdotter, M., Löken, L., Olausson, H., Vallbo, A., and Wessberg, J., 2009, Somatotopic organization of gentle touch processing in the posterior insular cortex. J Neurosci. Jul 22;29(29):9314-20.

24. Olausson, H., Lamarre, Y., Backlund, H., Morin, C., Wallin, B.G., Starck, G., Ekholm, S., Strigo, I., Worsley, K., Vallbo, A.B., and Bushnell, M.C., 2002, Unmyelinated tactile afferents signal touch and project to insular cortex. Nat Neurosci. Sep; 5(9): 900-4

25. Löken, L.S., Wessberg, J., Morrison, I., McGlone, F., and Olausson, H., 2009, Coding of pleasant touch by unmyelinated afferents in humans. Nat Neurosci. May;12(5):547-8. Epub 2009 Apr 12

26. Felton, D.L., and Józefowicz, R.F. (editors), 2003, Netter's Atlas of Human Neuroscience, 1st Ed. Icon Learning Systems

27. Melzack, R., 2001, Pain and the Neuromatrix in the Brain. Journal of Dental Education December 1, vol. 65no. 12 1378-1382

28. Saab, C.Y., Willis, W.D., 2003, The cerebellum: organization, functions and its role in nociception. Brain Res Brain Res Rev. Apr;42(1):85-95.

29. Moulton, E.A., Schmahmann, J.D., Becerra, L., and Borsook, D., 2010, The Cerebellum and Pain: Passive integrator or Active Participator? Brain Res Rev. Oct 5; 65(1): 14–27.

30. Hagains,C.E., Senapati, A.K., Huntington, P.J., He, J., Peng, Y.B., 2011, Inhibition of spinal cord dorsal horn activity by electrical stimulation of the cerebellar cortex. Journal of Neurophysiology. Nov. 1, Vol. 106 no. 5, 2515-2522.

31. Strata, P., 2015, The emotional cerebellum. Cerebellum. Oct; 14(5):570-7

32. Edin, B.B., and Johansson, N., 1995, Skin strain patterns provide kinaesthetic information to the human central nervous system. J Physiology 487.1 243-251

33. Collins, D.F., Refshauge, K.M, Todd, G., and Gandevia, S.C., 2005, Cutaneous receptors contribute to kinesthesia at the index finger, elbow, and knee. J Neurophysiol. Sep;94(3):1699-706

34. Proske, U., and Gandevia, S., 2009, The kinaesthetic senses. J Physiol 587.17 p. 4139–4146

35. Lundblad, L.C., Olausson, H.W., Malmeström, C., and Wasling, H.B., 2010, Processing in prefrontal cortex underlies tactile direction discrimination: An fMRI study of a patient with a traumatic spinal cord lesion. Neurosci Lett. Oct 15;483(3):197-200

36. Panek, I., Bui, T., Wright, A.T.B., and Brownstone, R.M., 2014, Cutaneous afferent regulation of motor function. Acta Neurobiol Exp. 74: 158–171

37. Foster, E., Wildner, H., Tudeau, L., Haueter, S., Ralvenius, W.T., Jegen, M., Johannssen, H., Hösli, L., Haenraets, K., Ghanem, A., Conzelmann, K., Bösl, M., and Zeilhofer, H.U., 2015, Targeted Ablation, Silencing, and Activation Establish Glycinergic Dorsal Horn Neurons as Key Components of a Spinal Gate for Pain and Itch. *Neuron*, 85: 1289-1304

38. Melzack, R., and Patrick D Wall, P.D., 1965, Pain Mechanisms: A New Theory. Science, New Series. Vol 150 No 3699 Nov 19 p971-979

39. Shechter, R., Baruch, K., Schwartz, M., and Rolls, A., 2011, Touch gives new life: mechanosensation modulates spinal cord adult neurogenesis. Mol Psychiatry. Mar;16(3):342-52

40. Kapitzke, D., Vetter, I., Cabot, P.J.; 2005, Endogenous opioid analgesia in peripheral tissues and the clinical implications for pain control. Ther Clin Risk Manag. Dec; 1(4): 279–297

41. Stein, C., Machelska, H.; Modulation of Peripheral Sensory Neurons by the Immune System: Implications for Pain Therapy. Pharmacological Reviews December 2011 vol. 63 no. 4860-881.

42. Stein, C., Schäfer, M., Machelska, H., 2003, Attacking Pain At Its Source: New Perspectives on Opioids. Nat Med. 2003;9(8)

43. Stein, C. 2000-2013, Opioid receptors on Peripheral Sensory Neurons. Madam Curie Bioscience Database. Landes Bioscience. Bookshelf ID: NBK6242 Retrieved May 15, 2016. http://www.ncbi.nlm.nih.gov/books/NBK6242/

44. Legrain V, Iannetti GD, Plaghki L, and Mouraux A., 2011, The pain matrix reloaded: a salience detection system for the body. Prog Neurobiol. Jan;93(1):111-24

45. Ossipov, M.H., 2009, Pain Pathways: Descending Modulation. Encyclopedia of Neuroscience, Larry R Squire (editor) Elsevier Ltd.

46. Chapman, C.R., Tuckett, R.P., and Song, C.W., 2008, Pain and Stress in a Systems Perspective: Reciprocal Neural, Endocrine and Immune Interactions. J Pain. Feb; 9(2): 122–145.

47. Dorko, B.L., 2003, The analgesia of movement: ideomotor activity and manual care. Journal of Osteopathic Medicine. 6(2): 93-95

48. Dorko, B.L., no date, The Characteristics of Correction. barrettdorko.com/articles/characte.htm , retrieved May 9, 2016

49. Rickards, L., Ideomotor Movement in Pain Management. Retrieved March 23 2016 from http://www.lukerickardsosteopath.net/ideomotor-movement-pain-management/

50. McCarthy, S., Rickards, L.D., Lucas, N., 2007, Using the concept of ideomotor therapy in the treatment of a patient with chronic neck pain: A single system research design. International Journal of Osteopathic Medicine. Dec., 10(4):104-112

5. NEURONS, NERVES, AND TUNNEL SYNDROMES

NEURONS: THEIR CARE AND FEEDING

Neurons are just like regular body cells, in that they have a nucleus, an interior, an exterior, and a membrane to separate outside from inside. The main difference is their *shape*: neurons are very long and very skinny, with *much* higher membrane to content ratio, with action potentials that can travel rapidly across, along, and about the whole organism, no matter how large. They are variable enough to serve creatures that vary in size from gnat to blue whale. From an exteroceptive input perspective, they are also the most mechanically excitable cells in the body.

Neurons are the longest cells in nerves, in the whole body. Neuroanatomist Jack Nolte describes a motor neuron to the big toe, as follows (paraphrased) – if the cell body were made the size of a tennis ball, the axon or the long skinny part would be a half-mile long and the size of a garden hose, and the dendrites would fill a small room (Ramachandran 2002). Now imagine a *sensory* neuron: a subset of these, i.e., large fast myelinated fibres, reach all the way up within dorsal pathways of the spinal cord to dorsal column nuclei - single cells that can span the distance between the skin on the end of your big toe and nuclei in your medulla (Mason 2011); staying within the metaphor, our *sensory* neuron is closer to a mile long (about 1.6 kilometers)!

Most of the fuel (25% for only 2% of the body's physicality!) consumed by the nervous system goes toward maintaining the receptor potential of this huge surface area of each neuronal cell, the all-important membrane, laden with receptors, so that action potentials can occur, then propagate (Felton et al. 2016).

Neurons have a lot more cell membrane to maintain than ordinary, blob-shaped body cells. To do their jobs, to keep those membranes ready to conduct an action potential, neurons burn a lot of metabolic energy in the form of glucose and oxygen – they need ample blood supply. Yet neurons must be protected from direct contact with blood (Rechthand and Rapoport 1987, Weerasuriya and

Mizisin 2011). Neuropathic pain may be linked to dysfunction in the blood nerve barrier (Lim et al. 2014, 2015).

Small thinly myelinated high threshold C-fibre sensory neurons innervate everything, including the coatings and layers and vessels of the nerves within which they travel. Most of their job, most of the time, is to lie quietly and exchange trophic factors with the tissues they innervate. Trophic factors from neurons are vital to tissue health. Trophic factors taken up *by* neurons from their target tissues (*neuro*trophic factors) are equally important for neuronal health (Zeliadt 2013, Mason 2011)). Every day of our lives, this trophic/neurotrophic exchange goes on everywhere in the body, like a cabbages-for-carrots swap economy.

It takes a lot to provoke nociceptive-capable C-fibres enough to make them mount an action potential, which is a good thing: their action potentials and substances *can* become entangled in physiological positive feedback loops of peripheral and central sensitization (Woolf 2011). However normal this operation may be for the nervous system, it can "*feel*" bad in terms of pain, perceived and having to be endured by the person living in and part of said nervous system. The brain may have to struggle for quite some time to attain appropriate descending modulation. Sometimes it just will not be able to, for genetic reasons or because of myriad other factors.

Neurons, because of the length of those axons, must transport substances to and from their membranes and target tissues for long distances, within their axoplasm. Any mechanical impairment of this transport system will affect the health of both the neuron and its target tissue. If neurons die, as in, for example, poorly controlled diabetes, target tissue also will die; organ failure and gangrene are serious complications of C-fibre death (Mason 2011).

NERVES: CONDUITS FOR NEURONS

Nerves are long, walled cylinders that protect neurons. Let us zoom inside a nerve: it is comprised of protective layers of connective tissue padding, within which neurons are contained inside smaller tubes called fascicles (A in the image depicted below), which can slide longitudinally, elongating a little bit, like telescopes, within the nerve (D). Fascicles are complexly branched however, not as straight as telescopes (B). Nerves are pierced through by vascular structure – remember, blood supply is the only way neurons can obtain all the oxygen and glucose they need to function properly (and remember that they need a lot) (B and C).

A. Neurons are grouped into bundles called fascicles, protected by connective tissue known as perineurium. Each neuron is protected by one or more Schwann cells

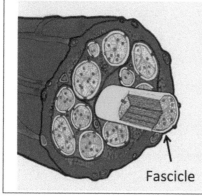

Fascicle

B. Fascicles are mainly longitudinal, but are highly branched, converging and diverging within the nerve

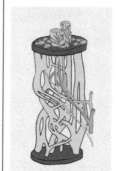

C. Nerves are well supplied with blood through regional vessels, which penetrate within the fascicles to supply neurons and their cell coats, Schwann cells

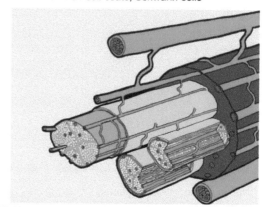

D. Fascicles can telescope in and out through nerves a certain amount, with normal movment and exercise, action which pulls attached vessels and stimulates them.
As long as there is movement variety, of short duration, such elongation does no harm and helps keep nerves slidey and healthy

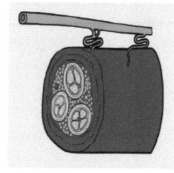 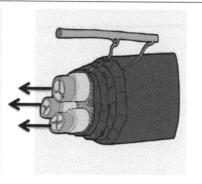

Images adapted from Lundborg (1988) and Gilroy (2012): A) Anatomy of a peripheral nerve; epineurium (green), perineurium (turquoise) forms the fascicle of grouped neurons, endoneurium and Schwann cells (dark pink), neurons (yellow: B) Fascicular branching within a nerve, vasa nervorum and nervi nervorum: C) Vessel attached to nerve, penetrating as deep as the endoneurium: D) Fascicular sliding within nerve allows it to elongate, moves the attached vasculature.

Nerve layers are innervated by some of the neurons within them (see Image B). Neurons that innervate a nerve are referred to as nervi nervorum (Bove 2008). The vasculature within a nerve is vasa nervorum (Adams 1942). The neural array to vasculature within a nerve is nervi vasorum. The blood supply to the walls of blood vessels is the vasa vasorum.

All arterial blood vessels, except those of capillary size, have walls filled with smooth muscle cells that are under strict neural control, mainly by the sympathetic nervous system, via efferent C-fibres, to manage moment-by-moment adaptations for stable blood pressure. They also are innervated by nociceptive-capable afferent C fibres. Capillaries are exempt from innervation as their mechanism for blood flow is via passive capillary action.

DermoNeuroModulating | Diane Jacobs

Veins and arteries are connected to nerves, throughout every inch of their 72 kilometers, by thin regional vessels (Lundborg 1988). Vessels are of widely varying size, and must traverse through layers of body wall also, together with nerves they serve.

Getting blood through small thin regional vessels into and out of nerve is somewhat perilous, as the vascular system may be pulled in slightly different directions than the nerves it supplies. If a nerve does not receive adequate blood supply because of mechanical tension affecting regional vessels feeding it, or it becomes backed up and compressed from within from mechanical tension affecting regional vessels that drain it, its own nociceptive innervation may activate.

A tunnel syndrome is basically a cranky nerve whose tunnel has become a compressive or tensional danger to the neurons inside it (Lundborg 1988); nociceptive neurons embedded within the nerve walls that confine them (Bove 2008) signal "danger." Tunnel syndromes of a non-medical kind may arise because of too much movement of a repetitive kind, or simply not enough movement of any kind. (Couch potatoes, look out.) Nociceptive neurons within a nerve, complaining, activate others nearby, to create a so-called sterile inflammation or peripheral sensitization, i.e., "neuritis" inside nerve itself (IASP taxonomy page).

One must comprehend the several orders of magnitude and scale involved here. Every neuron, no matter how tiny, depends on the supply of oxygen and glucose entering its containment fascicle, surrounded by tough perineurium, via capillaries of appropriately tiny size, and drainage vessels to take away the substances it makes and exports to its local environment.

Neurons, and the Schwann cells that enclose them, are very active metabolically. Metabolites must be continuously flushed away to prevent noxious build-up that could trip chemo-sensitive nociceptors over their threshold. (By way of analogy consider what happens to the skin of a baby who has been left in a wet diaper for too long a time.) Nerves have only partial lymphatic drainage (Volpi 2013), so venous drainage is crucial.

What is amazing is that this very basic, fine-grained interactive physiological system works as well as it does *inside* enclosed nerve layers and wrappings, most of the time. A classic primary inflammatory response, complete with peripheral sensitization, can occur within the enclosed space of a nerve. This can increase nociceptive input rather abruptly and intensely.

Keep in mind what spinal cords do if barraged by nociceptive input.

Now let us zoom back out, and look at the peripheral neurovascular system *in situ*: a forest of vascular and neural branches and twigs exists, embedded within a complex multi-cellular organism. Neurons and vessels must supply every bit of tissue, including their *own* wrappings, with innervation and danger surveillance on behalf of the *organism as a whole;*

1. so that all cells in all tissues of every kind may receive innervation, oxygen, and all other important messenger substances from the brain, like the hormones that blood carries about, and;

2. so that their cell secretions, excretions, and metabolic messages are carried to other cells far away to be utilized, or destroyed and discarded by the organism as a whole.

Conjoined and co-dependent at every size scale throughout the entire body, this forest of physiological tubing slides against structural layers and through tunnels and across joints as the organism moves about. All of this must occur uninterruptedly even as they are tugged at, moved, and elongated by the slide and glide of their attached and moving containment system. Slack and spiraled, loose and forgiving, the containment system will usually allow physiological function to occur everywhere in any position. Vessels in nerves and nerves themselves are mechanosensitive; tugging stimulates blood flow into and out of nerves, and helps keep the neurovascular bundle, and our tissues, and us, healthy. Exercise helps keep it all healthy and optimal. Motion is lotion. However, if the tugging is not varied enough, is repetitive or sustained too long or is insufficient, there can be consequences. If and when nociceptive neurons within nerves sensitize and activate as part of an inflammatory process, nerves themselves can produce important nociceptive input contributions that can eventually lead to a pain experience (Bove and Light 1997), without there ever having had to be any overt "injury" or "tissue damage" to speak of. Peripheral sensitization can make normal tugging of neural tunnel on nerve "hurt," sometimes so much that ordinary movement becomes impossible.

NEURAL TUNNELS AND MECHANICAL DEFORMATION

Have you ever taken a cross-country road trip? Highways traverse varied landscape: some parts of the highway might be wide and soft and forgiving with broad shoulders, while in other parts the road might narrow to single-lane to cross a bridge or to wind perilously around a rocky outcropping.

Nerve tunnels are far from regular, even at the best of times. Think of a neural tunnel as a tubular highway.

As a peripheral nerve courses along, its tunnel could be through usually forgiving, easily deformable and relaxed soft tissue. Other parts of the tunnel might force the nerve to have to squeeze through an interosseous membrane between bones, or through holes in bones, or between thick tendons, or through a grommet hole in a tough sheet of fascia, then have to slide against the edge at a sharp angle in an abrupt change of direction, or branch at a very wide angle, all of which will make a nerve much more vulnerable to mechanical deformation. Anatomical variations might result in a nerve branching oddly in a vulnerable location, and being more deformable at that branch point.

TUNNEL SYNDROMES AND PATHODYNAMICS

Pathodynamics co-occur with tunnel syndromes (Lundborg 1988, 1988; Pećina, Krmpotić-Nemanić, and Markiewitz 2001), and often accompany complaints of emergent or persisting regional pain (Treed 2008). The word 'pathodynamics' implies merely that a nerve cannot, for whatever reason, seem to move normally within its tunnels.

A pathodynamic problem may be inferred from complaints of pain accompanied by limited movement. It may be putatively confirmed by the presence of carefully examined and ascertained small barriers to passive movement of a patient's body part by a therapist, and/or accompanying symptoms as reported by the patient.

Tunnel syndromes themselves may arise due to a pathological condition, or may be temporary consequence of some form of behaviour, which can be altered. The tunnels, through which nerves must slide, have outsides and insides. Looking at a tunnel from the perspective of the nerve, there are only two possibilities:

1. *Tunnel restriction from outside the nerve*: the nerve is normal, but the tunnel surrounding it has become narrowed because of some external factor. There may be a) pathological reasons such as pressure from a tumor or a fracture, or b) non-pathological reasons such as persistent mechanical deformation caused by habits or behaviour; consequent defensive spinal cord adaptation has ostensibly led to chronic efferent tensioning, to both striate and smooth muscle cells, resulting in motor output holding patterns.

2. *Tunnel restriction from within the nerve*: the tunnel is normal, but the nerve that slides through it has swollen and no longer easily fits the tunnel. There may be a) pathological reasons such as pressure from something, e.g., a neuroma, or thickening in nerve wall secondary to an inflammatory process ("neuritis"), or b) non-pathological reasons such as impairment in the drainage of intraneural circulation, secondary to mechanical deformation caused by behaviour, either resting or repetitive.

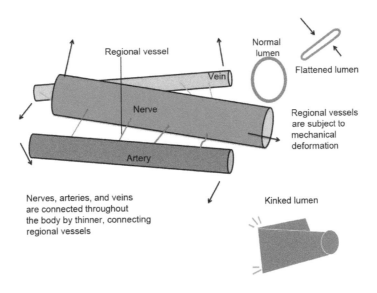

Normal movement assists nerve circulation physiology. If regional vessels become kinked, or stretched and narrowed, or flattened, blood flow to and from a nerve will be impaired. There is usually enough redundant circulation that no neuron will starve or drown, under normal conditions, with plenty of daily activity, and variety of activity. Nerve walls are innervated by nociceptive-capable fibres that report to the CNS about changes in local internal milieu from prolonged mechanical deformation.

Two excellent sources of information regarding tunnel syndromes that were used to develop DNM are Lundborg (1988) and Pećina, Krmpotić-Nemanić, and Markiewitz (2001).

Göran Lundborg

Lundborg, an orthopaedic surgeon, was dissatisfied with the knowledge base in his field as it pertained to nerve injury and repair. He had come to realize that surgery to fixate bone, no matter how brilliant, would be in vain if the patient woke up unable to use their beautifully repaired limb because the nerves in it had died from hypoxia secondary to the blood pressure cuff restriction necessary during surgery to maintain a bloodless field. He spent much of the 1970's and 1980's working with rabbits and painstakingly working out nerve movement and physiology and how these related. His goal was to establish time parameters: how long could blood pressure cuffs be left on before nerve health was endangered? How long could one operate before cuffs needed to be released to allow nerves to perfuse and their function to recover? He found problems with the cuffs themselves – what the pressure gauge indicated was not always the actual pressure delivered by the equipment – he managed to persuade cuff companies to standardize calibration more accurately. His book, Nerve Injury and Repair (1988) is a great story, and contains the best illustrations of how nerves and neurons respond to mechanical stresses that I have ever seen.

Regarding tunnel syndromes, Lundborg concluded that:

1. Localized microvascular interference and structural changes in a nerve or its adjacent tissues can lead to nerve compression syndromes
2. Tissues subjected to pressure will deform and create pressure gradients; compressed (neural) tissue becomes redistributed toward areas of lower pressure
3. At sites where nerves pass through tight tunnels formed by stiff tissue boundaries, they can develop compression syndromes

Lundborg's main interest was carpal tunnel syndrome. However, there are 72 kilometers of nerve and *all* of them have tunnels to contend with. Any nerve can become compromised in any tunnel, and will be especially vulnerable at branch points.

Tunnel Syndromes: the book

In the book, Tunnel Syndromes: Peripheral Nerve Compression Syndromes, Pećina *et al.* 2001 develop a bigger picture with documented descriptions of *more than 50* distinct, medically recognized tunnel syndromes; it is also well worth buying. The authors put forth the following points, which I have paraphrased (and added supplemental comments and references in italics, in brackets):

1. Tunnel syndromes can occur from external pressure on nerves from within the body; e.g., a tumour pressing into a nerve, etc.. Many are "idiopathic," however, which means no obvious

cause such as a tumour. *(As therapists, we might consider mechanical deformation, secondary to misuse or disuse of the body, as a possible, plausible, possibly ubiquitous contributing factor, in the case of "idiopathic" tunnel syndromes.)*

2. Function of a nerve can be dramatically altered without compromise of outside space such as external pressure on a tunnel: medical and other conditions can adversely affect nerve function, such as:

   · Inflammatory changes that thicken a neural wall and reduce blood supply

   · Oedema in nerves or nerve container secondary to hormonal changes from pregnancy, menopause, birth control pills, hypothyroidism/myxedema

   · Anatomical variations coupled with ordinary movement or repetitive movement

   · *(To this list I would add diabetes and accompanying changes in blood osmolality that interferes with nerve nutrition; see Mason 2011)*

   (Thickened nerves make for pathodynamics within narrower parts of their tunnels.)

3. Ischemic changes first affect sensory fibres; if they continue motor fibres will be affected *(Supported by Hofmeijer et al. 2013. This is important in dermoneuromodulation reasoning, which recognizes the relevance of cutaneous nerves and cutaneous rami containing sensory fibres, clinical navigating by the relieving of hyperalgesia/"sore spots," avoiding areas of frank allodynia, and in general, doing one's best to avoid adding any more nociception to an already sensitized nervous system.)*

4. Pain is the most common symptom *(there is usually still plenty of time to turn things around at this stage)*

5. Anatomic variations create restricted mobility for a nerve between its origin and its course through its tunnel *(there is nothing we as therapists can do, directly, about anatomical variation. It is part of the uncertainty to be embraced. We might bear it in mind, however, as a possible contributing factor, and remind ourselves that the nervous system can adapt to nearly anything if given a low enough slope in terms of time and regular spaced practice of new motor output.)*

6. X-rays do not show soft tissue variations, which can be compressive factors in many cases *(See point 5.)*

7. A nerve that abruptly enters a new tissue produces a fulcrum on which external forces can act *(cutaneous nerves containing fascicles with only sensory and autonomic motor neurons travel further and have one more tough fascial body wall to pierce through, and branch distally from, often at extreme angles; see Lundborg's conclusions, point 3)*

Consider the challenge faced by neurons that must span segments of body and limb that have huge ranges of movement. Nerves *can* and usually *will* adapt to almost anything physical that humans can come up with, but it takes time, patience, and careful, judiciously spaced and paced practice before they can handle it, without unnecessarily provoking the central nervous system: meanwhile the central nervous system must learn that provocation by sensory neurons does not usually signal harm, even though it may *feel* like "danger;" as Butler has pointed out, hurt does not equal harm (Butler 2000).

NEURODYNAMICS

The term encompasses both a description of normal movement of nerves in the body, and a manual therapy concept (Shacklock 1995) based on all the new information about the care and feeding of the peripheral nervous system that emerged based on Lundborg's work and the work of others. The locus of concern in manual therapy moved away from trying to "fix" "joints" and joint-based 'faulty' biomechanics, etc., to consideration of nerve and nervous system and nerve pathodynamics. This was wonderful evolution in my opinion; I regard with enormous appreciation the pioneers who initiated it, and those who have studied and popularized it over the last 30 years. Neurodynamics as therapy represents excellent advance in the world of manual therapy, mostly by making therapeutic handling of someone else's body more refined, less nociceptive.

Shacklock made a short ultrasound video (Shacklock 2015) that depicts a long deep median nerve moving normally within the arm by bending the hand back and forth. He then moves his head into side flexion away and toward, and the nerve moves independently from the tendons, which represent the neural container and lie relaxed. His video provided proof of concept that it is possible to move deep nerves from outside the body, to move a nerve longitudinally either way through its tunnel by moving either the distal part of its container into which it is cutaneously embedded, or the proximal end, by moving the spinal column. Recently Shacklock et. al. (2016) showed that passive contralateral nerve movement can be obtained as well.

MOVEMENT THERAPY

We want our patients to be able to move better after treating them manually, and to *practice* moving, because movement of nerves – judicious, spaced, regular, and on-going movement therapy, is what will help with pain in the long run.

Manual treatment will usually help improve pain and movement, but only in the short term. Movement therapy such as deliberate neural gliding – care and feeding of nerve through movement - is important in the first three days following treatment. Movement therapy should be easy and convenient to do in any position or environment, and take only a few short moments. I propose it be done every couple hours, only 4 or 5 repetitions. You could frame it as "taking a move-better pill" (credited to Neil Pearson, who mentioned this at a pain conference in 2014) at constant spaced intervals (e.g., every two or three hours) over the first 3 days following a session. Receptors will be replaced on neurons and by day four, any improvement subsequently practiced can be considered optimally stabilized and any gain secured. Movement therapy can be reduced to a few times a day after that for a few days or weeks longer. Establishing a new habit of checking in on how one's body feels is important - it is just too easy to simply ignore it until such time as it is too late.

If you want to feel better in a body, learn to feel your body better

Simple brisk daily walking is good for getting blood all through nerves, and for maintaining the ability of inherent mechanisms to get blood through nerves. Taking stairs instead of elevator is good for maintaining foot, leg, pelvis and low back nerves.

Floor work is very beneficial for back nerves. It is good for humans to remain good friends with the floor, throughout life, by visiting the floor on a regular basis, getting down and lying on it. Getting down and up off the floor is in itself good mobility exercise.

Floors are hard, flat, inert, level, and even.

They do not change.

They do not vary.

Whatever you "feel" when you lie on the floor will be all about you, not about the floor.

When you first lie down, you may feel parts of yourself pressing in too hard or not even touching - that is an indication of tension. Take a mental snapshot of the topographical map you can "feel" with the weight of your body resting against the floor.

It does not much matter what you *do* on the floor – any mild movement suggestion found on YouTube, such as Feldenkrais, or Somatics™, will do. Make up your own movements if you wish. Learn how to let go of tension by moving parts of yourself, thoughtfully, deeply breathing and exhaling, lengthening (telescoping) through one side of your body, or diagonally, lengthening your arms, and/or legs, one by one or all at once, whatever you want to try. Be creative. Your movement does not need to look beautiful, it only needs to be effective, and therefore *feel* beautiful.

At the end, check the map you made in the beginning. It will likely feel flatter, like more of you is *in contact with* the floor, like you have softened and widened and lengthened. You might notice fewer places feeling like they are digging into the floor, or maybe if some still are, pressing not nearly as hard.

If you become fond of the floor, you *may* become adventuresome enough to even try a bit of yoga. People who are even more adventuresome may decide to join a gym and start lifting. People who are socially inclined may want to take up a team sport.

REFERENCES

1. Ramachandran, V.S., (Editor), 2002, Encyclopedia of the Human Brain, Four-Volume Set. Academic Press; 1 edition July 10. Jack Nolte quoted by Jay B. Angevine Jr., p. 335, in chapter, "Nervous System, Organization of," p.313

2. Mason, P., (Author), 2011, Medical Neurobiology. Oxford University Press, USA; 1 edition May 19

3. Felten, D., O'Banion, M.K., and Maida, M.S., (editors), 2016, Netter's Atlas of Neuroscience. Elsevier; 3rd edition

4. Rechthand, E., and Rapoport, S.I., 1987, Regulation of the microenvironment of peripheral nerve: Role of the blood-nerve barrier. Progress in Neurobiology Vol 28 p 303-343

5. Weerasuriya, A., and Mizisin, A.P., 2011, The blood-nerve barrier: structure and functional significance. Methods Mol Biol. 686:149-73

6. Lim, T.K., Shi, X.Q., Martin, H.C., Huang, H., Luheshi, G., Rivest, S., and Zhang, J., 2014, Blood-nerve barrier dysfunction contributes to the generation of neuropathic pain and allows targeting of injured nerves for pain relief. Pain. May;155(5):954-67

7. Lim, T.K., Shi, X.Q., Johnson, J.M., Rone, M.B., Antel, J.P., David, S., and Zhang, J., 2015, Peripheral Nerve Injury Induces Persistent Vascular Dysfunction and Endoneurial Hypoxia, Contributing to the Genesis of Neuropathic Pain. The Journal of Neuroscience, 25 February, 35(8): 3346-3359

8. Zeliadt, N., 2013, Rita Levi-Montalcini: NGF, the protypical growth factor. Proc Natl Acad Sci U S A. 2013 Mar 26; 110(13): 4873–4876.

9. Woolf, C.J., 2011, Central sensitization: Implications for the diagnosis and treatment of pain. Pain. Mar; 152(3 Suppl): S2–15.

10. Lundborg, G. (author), 1988, Nerve Injury and Repair. New York. Churchill Livingstone

11. Gilroy, A.M., MacPherson, B.R., Ross L.M., Schuenke, M., Erik Schulte, E., and Schumacher, U. (authors) 2012, Atlas of Anatomy 2nd ed. Thieme

12. Bove, G., 2008, Epi-Perineurial Anatomy, Innervation, and Axonal Nociceptive Mechanisms. J Bodyw Mov Ther. Jul; 12(3): 185–190.

13. Adams, W.E., 1942, The Blood Supply of Nerves - Historical Review J Anat. Jul. 76(Pt 4): 323–341.

14. Lundborg, G., 1988, Intraneural microcirculation. Orthop Clin North Am. Jan;19(1):1-12.

15. Note regarding "Neuritis", IASP taxonomy page, http://www.iasp-pain.org/Taxonomy#Peripheralneuropathicpain

16. Volpi,N., Guarna, M., Lorenzoni, P., Franci, D., Massai, L., and Grasso, G., 2013, Characterization of lymphatic vessels in human peripheral neuropathies. Italian Journal of Anatomy and Embryology, [S.l.], p. 12, Feb. ISSN 2038-5129.

17. Bove, G.M., and Light, A.R., 1997, The nervi nervorum: Missing link for neuropathic pain? The Journal of Pain Autumn Vol 6 Issue 3 P 181-190

18. Pećina, M.M., Krmpotić-Nemanić, J., and Markiewitz, A.D. (authors), 2001, Tunnel Syndromes. CRC Press; 3 edition August 16

19. Treed, R.D., Jensen, T.S., Campbell, J.N., Cruccu, G., Dostrovsky, J.O., Griffin, J.W., Hansson, P., Hughes, R., Nurmikko, T., and Serra, K., 2008, Neuropathic pain: redefinition and a grading system for clinical and research purposes. Neurology Apr 29; 70 (18): 1630-5

20. Hofmeijer, J., Franssen, H., van Schelven, L.J., and van Putten, M.J.A.M., 2013, Why Are Sensory Axons More Vulnerable for Ischemia than Motor Axons? PLoS One 8(6): e67113.

21. Butler, D.S. (Author), 2000, Sensitive Nervous System. Noigroup Publications; 1 edition January 1

22. Shacklock, M. 1995, Neurodynamics. Physiotherapy, Jan. Vol 81 No 1 p9-16

23. Shacklock, M., 2015, Nerve movement in 2015 - 20th Anniversary of neurodynamics in physical and manual therapy. Neurodynamic Solutions newsletter, Dec

24. Shacklock, M., Yee, B., Van Hoof, T., Foley, R., Boddie, K., Lacey, E., Poley, J.,B., Rade, M., Kankaanpää, M., Kröger, H., Airaksinen, O., 2016, Slump Test: Effect of Contralateral Knee Extension on Response Sensations in Asymptomatic Subjects and Cadaver Study. Spine (Phila Pa 1976)Feb;41(4):E205-10

6. TREATING TUNNEL SYNDROMES BY MOVING NERVES AND SKIN

THE SKIN ORGAN AND CUTANEOUS RAMI

Nash et al. (2004) described how the skin organ is held against the body by thousands of small skin ligaments, which explains why an organ that weighs as much as the skeleton can feel weightless. They stated that many skin ligaments are hollow and convey neural structure to the skin surface. Hollow ones conveying neural structure would equate to being cutaneous rami neural tunnels. But what did they look like? Their paper did not provide much visual information that was of any use to me as a manual therapist.

I could not find *any* images in any of the common anatomy books available to me that visually depicted how cutaneous nerves disseminated into the skin organ. In 2006 a librarian helped me do a search for papers, but even with access to numerous databases he could only find about 15 papers, most of them by plastic surgeons, mostly about preserving cutaneous rami in breasts and faces, illustrated with crude diagrams only, and most of them not available in English.

In 2007 the anatomy lab at University of British Columbia kindly allowed me in to dissect a cadaver arm in order to visualize these small nerves, and even relaxed their policy to give me permission to photograph them.

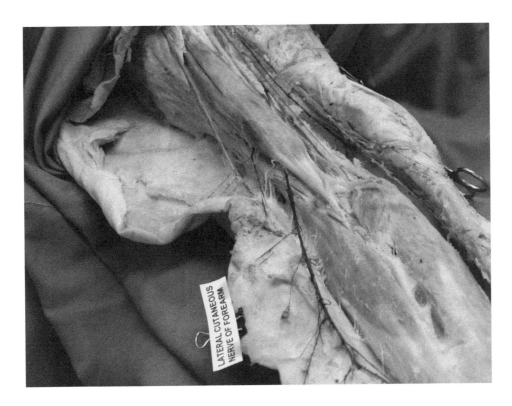

Photo by Diane Jacobs 2007: Dissection exposure of the lateral cutaneous nerve of the arm with rami intact. Subcutaneous fat has been carefully removed. Neural structure including tubular skin ligament structure conveying neural rami to the surface have been rendered visible by darkening with a felt pen.

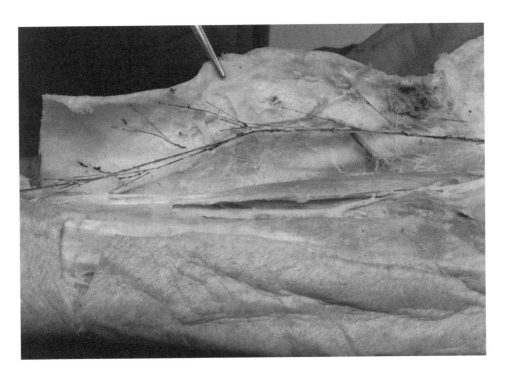

Photo by Diane Jacobs 2007: Same dissection, view from medial side of arm.

Cutaneous nerves are longer than motor nerves; there are many more kilometers of fascicles that contain these than there are fascicles containing motor neurons, whose journeys end when they embed into striate muscle closer to the center axis of the body. If we add the combined length of all their disseminating rami, cutaneous nerves are longer still.

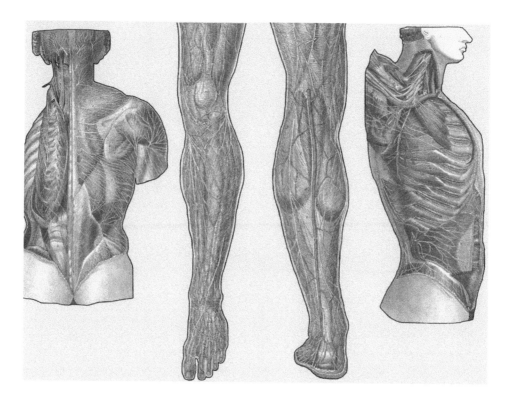

Images from AnatomyAtlases.org by permission. Cutaneous nerves (yellow) are everywhere, traveling just beneath or within the skin organ.

Additionally and importantly, cutaneous nerve branches also disseminate inward to help innervate the dense fascial wall, through which they pierce, and also tendons and aponeuroses that lie beneath the skin organ (Stilwell 1957, 1957; O'Brien 1992; Doral et al. 2010; Uquillas et al. 2015).

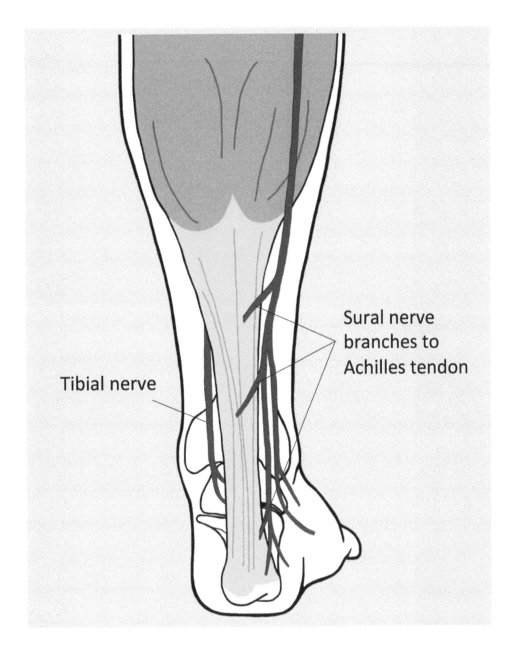

Adapted from Uquillas et al. 2015: Sural nerve rami bend inward to help innervate outer surface of Achilles tendon. Tibial nerve rami innervate it from behind.

Do cutaneous nerves have tunnel syndromes?

Yes, they do; e.g., there is a named condition called "meralgia paresthetica" which means "thigh pain", and is an entrapment of the lateral cutaneous nerve of the thigh. Another named condition known as "notalgia paresthetica" describes entrapment of a cutaneous dorsal ramus (Pećina et al 2001). In the 1980's and 1990's Robert Maigne, an MD in France, published several papers (most of them in French) on putative entrapment syndromes of long dorsal rami that form cutaneous nerves over buttocks and lateral pelvis (Maigne and Maigne 1991). William Applegate (Applegate 2002) has described abdominal cutaneous nerve entrapment as a syndrome, and a commonly overlooked cause of abdominal pain. However most cutaneous nerve entrapments still lack distinct names.

Anywhere that pain is felt in some body part, coupled with a tender point located where the cutaneous nerve supplying the skin of that region predictably exits from deeper layers, consider trying to affect it favourably by targeting the exit point with an unloading manouver. You can get your hands on skin organ directly, and by moving it, move the entire neural array contained and embedded within it, easily. You can combine skin pull with body position, and unload hyperalgesic tender points such that they stop feeling tender, which in turn, *may* help the *entire* nervous system change its output to one less "painful."

MOVING NERVES THERAPEUTICALLY

How does DNM differ from Neurodynamics?

Both consider nerves and movement of nerves as main treatment focus; however DNM takes it a little bit further:

1. **Quadruped position**: The mammalian peripheral nervous system evolved in quadrupeds. The neural container in any given area might be widened, softened, shortened, deliberately, by quadruped positioning, then adding skin traction or ballooning for even more unloading of nerve.

2. **Consideration of skin**: The skin organ is regarded as a fabulously easy-to-access, deformable, heavily-innervated, neurologically primed and loaded *handle*, toward which a patient's awareness may be directed, by which one might physically affect peripheral nerves toward favourable outcome and affect the nervous system as a whole.

3. **Consideration of cutaneous nerves**: Principles of neurodynamics are extended to include possible elongating longitudinal slide of *specific fascicles* within the nerve itself, namely those that contain only sensory and autonomic motor neurons, that branch off the main nerve in relatively predictable locations to supply the skin organ.

4. **Consideration of cutaneous rami**: Cutaneous nerves supplying the skin organ, and their rami, are included in clinical reasoning as being as deserving of consideration as any deeply buried nerve trunk; also considered is whether or not there may be a relationship between therapeutically applied movement of their multiple rami, and pain relief.

5. **Movement may be applied to nerves in/from any direction**: Consideration is given to how rotational forces might be applied to nerves, or to their cutaneous rami, longitudinally ('twizzling' – see below), or simply how deeper nerves may be bent or bowed locally within their deformable container from, and at, any angle.

6. **Blood flow while treating**: Drainage of blood flow out of nerve is considered to be just as important as blood flow into, from a mechanical standpoint; effort is made to imagine how to *not* impede blood flow while treating, how one might ostensibly promote it instead, by *un*loading nerve instead of loading it more, creating conditions for less rather than more hypoxia and adverse mechanical deformation.

7. **Self-correction by the nervous system**: More emphasis in placed on nervous system *self-correction*, how to recognize it while it is happening, and how to wait until it feels complete in one area before moving on to another area.

INTRODUCING "TWIZZLE"

Clinical reasoning around a specific pain presentation:

Let us look at a pain situation, one that is relatively common: the patient complains of "pain" in the buttock, a stabbing kind, felt on movement, which does not move or spread. It might be associated with limited straight leg raise, but there is no leg pain or paresthesia. It gets better or worse but never goes away. On palpation, there *is* accompanying hyperalgesia, but it seems to be quite deep in the buttock. History and symptoms do not correspond to this pain being related in any way to the sciatic nerve, but it *could* be some other motor nerve deep in there, that has become hyperalgesic. How might we approach *this* problem from a dermoneuromodulating, neurodynamic perspective?

1. Clearly, moving the local skin will be much less effective if cutaneous nerves are not directly involved.

2. We choose to *not* assume that some deep muscle (e.g., piriformis) is misbehaving, then take aim and apply direct pressure with the point of an elbow, try to stretch it mechanically from without and hope for the best. That adds more nociceptive load to the nervous system which may result in even more guarding by the spinal cord, and perpetuation of the pain problem. Remember, in this treatment framework, muscle tension is not defect, it is nervous system defense.

3. It does not seem to be the sciatic nerve, so the more conventional longitudinal neurodynamic strategy usually targeted to the sciatic nerve, i.e., bending and straightening of knee with dorsi and plantarflexion of foot in a sitting position, is not as likely to be effective.

We do want to do something that will be immediately effective. So what *can* we do? We have to use our brain, remember the anatomy, physiology, and movment of nerves, what nerves need in life, apply clinical reasoning and try to unload the nerve *indirectly*. *But how?*

A new neurodynamic concept — Twizzling

We know that nerves are slidey inside containers. We cannot be sure which way the nerve *needs* to move or be moved, but luckily we work with usually conscious patients with whom we can interact verbally. All we need to assume is that nerve and container have relative movement, and all we need to do is move nerve and container one way or another, and ask the patient which way results in relief, for them.

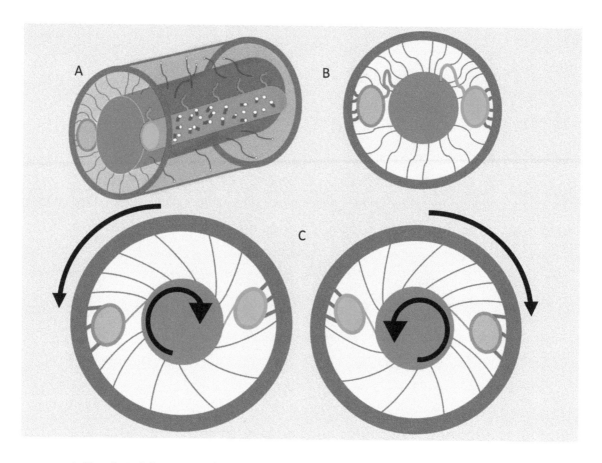

A. Hypothetical short section of nerve with its accompanying vessels, suspended on all sides by fibres which permit longitudinal sliding movement of the nerve within the neural container and lengthening of attached vascular regional vessels. B. If vessels are more firmly attached to the wall of the container than the nerve (C and D), then relative rotational torque forces may be introduced between nerve and neural container; mechanical forces will tend to converge on the regional vessels that enter nerve.

Patient prone: flex hip and knee off side of table

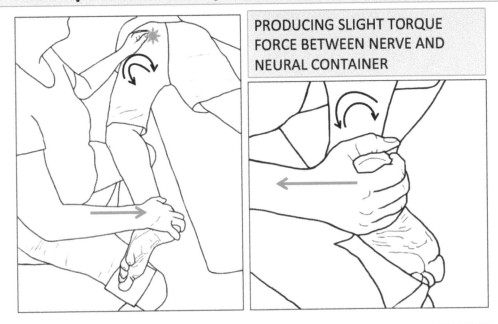

PRODUCING SLIGHT TORQUE FORCE BETWEEN NERVE AND NEURAL CONTAINER

SHORTEN AND WIDEN NEURAL CONTAINERS: BLOCK KNEE, TWIZZLE NERVE/CONTAINER BY ROTATING FOOT EITHER WAY

Treatment concept: Leg represents neural container. With hip and knee flexed, the container is short-ened and widened. Using the patient's foot as the handle, leg can be rotated one way or the other to produce relative motion between nerve and container and affect branches of the neural tree lying much more proximal, regardless of not knowing precise direction in which target nerve disseminates. One asks the patient to choose which way that they feel results in more decrease in hyperalgesia, for them.

SUMMARY OF NEURODYNAMIC TREATMENT CONCEPTS IN DNM

1. Twizzling (described above)

2. Nerves, and their attached vascular within neural tunnels, may be moved in any direction or combination of directions.

> **Even if you cannot touch or move deep nerves directly, you can move three-tube systems and their containers in different directions, and affect them indirectly**

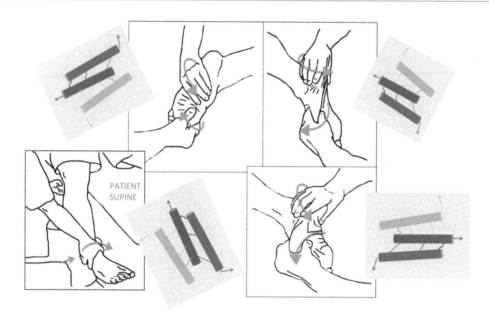

Three D Movement

3. Quadruped position whenever possible, including treatment in sidelying with hips, knees flexed.

NERVOUS SYSTEM
EVOLVED IN QUADRUPED
POSITION (LIMBS FLEXED
AT TRUNK)

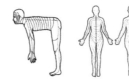

TREATMENT IN QUADRUPED POSITION TO SHORTEN AND
WIDEN NEURAL CONTAINER

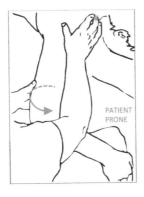

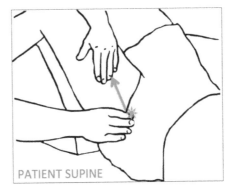

CUTANEOUS NERVES AT
SHOULDER TREATED IN PRONE,
ARM OFF SIDE OF BED, FLEXED

CUTANEOUS NERVES AT HIP
TREATED IN SUPINE, LEGS FLEXED
OVER BOLSTER

Bringing the body into a flexed position will usually promote more comfort and relaxation

4. Moving skin in any direction.

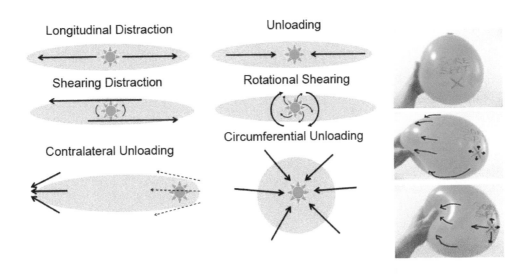

Skin organ is like a diving suit, a thick, rubbery layer than can be deformed in any direction. Pulling
skin away from a sore spot will decrease its tenderness way better than pushing into it.

5. Moving cutaneous rami.

By moving skin one moves cutaneous rami slightly in their tubular skin ligament tunnels:

One can balloon skin to shorten and widen cutaneous neural tunnels:

BASIC BALLOON PHYSICS: All the layers of body wall, and anything inside them, are attached to each other, while still allowing for some slide between

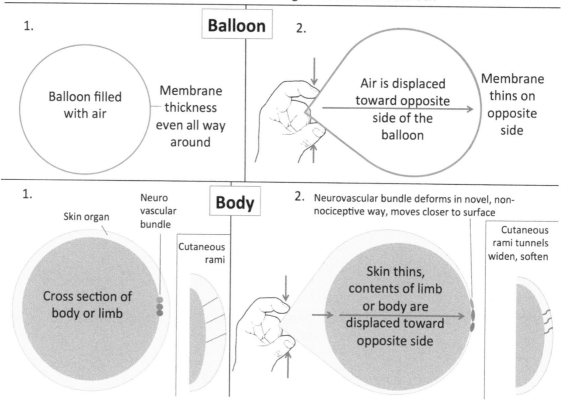

One can grasp non-hyperalgesic areas of skin opposite side of limb or trunk exhibiting tenderness, take up available slack; a) contents will move toward hyperalgesic side; b) skin organ will be pulled multidirectionally away from tender area; c) neural containers of cutaneous rami may be widened and shortened. You could think of skin as a balloon. On a person, the membrane is not enclosing air, but it will be enclosing all sorts of tissues that will easily displace to the opposite side from where you are grasping or moving skin surface. Below skin, you will be moving and thereby affecting, neural structure, both superficial and deep.

6. Balloon approach to favourably deform deeper nerves passing through tunnels at large joints:

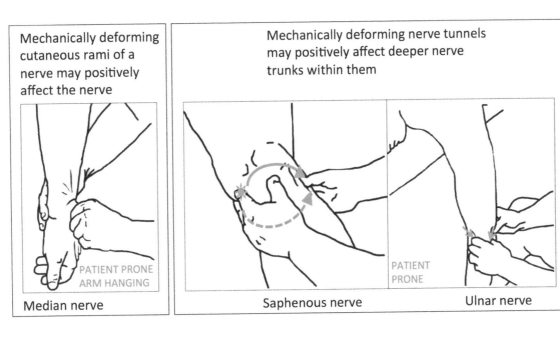

Neural tunnels are distorted by being dragged laterally in two simultaneous horizontal directions by skin bal-looning approach. Deliberate mechanical deformation of the skin organ overlying and connected to neural tunnels can tug vascular supply of cutaneous rami and deeper nerve trunks in novel and relieving ways.

Clinical note: If a person's skin is shiny or dry or slippery, you can use a hand-sized piece of dycem to gain better traction. Dycem is great for this task – it is sticky, light, and can be washed and dried easily between clients, making it infinitely reuseable.

SUMMARY

There is no direct scientific evidence yet, to either strengthen or negate these particular treatment elaborations. We are working with ideas only at this point, plausible within a framework of interacting with the nervous system, biopsychosocially, physically, functionally and physiologically. It might be useful to remember that delivering of innocuous mechanical input in the context of grooming is common among vertebrates of all kinds. Primates advanced this behaviour into the social sphere. I believe manual therapy in *human* primates is simply evolved social grooming, is inherently motivated in our human vertebrate brains and our primate species. Maybe it does not need evidence, just some science-based reframing, and acceptance on that basis (Jacobs D 2011, Jacobs D and Silvernail J 2011, Morrison et al 2011, Øberg, Normann, Gallagher 2015).

REFERENCES

1. Nash, L.G., Phillips, M.N., Nicholson, H., Barnett, R., and Zhang, M., 2004, Skin Ligaments: Regional distribution and morphology. Clinical Anatomy. Vol 17 Issue 4 p 287-293

2. Stilwell, D.L., 1957, Regional variations in the innervation of deep fasciae and aponeuroses. The Anatomical Record Volume 127, Issue 4, pages 635–653, April

3. Stilwell, D.L., 1957, The innervation of tendons and aponeuroses. American Journal of Anatomy Volume 100, Issue 3, pages 289–317, May

4. O'Brien, M., 1992, Functional anatomy and physiology of tendons. Clin Sports Med. Jul;11(3):505-20

5. Doral, M.N., Alam, M., Bozkurt, M., Turhan, E., Atay, O.A., Dönmez, G., and Maffulli, N., 2010, Functional anatomy of the Achilles tendon. Knee Surg Sports Traumatol Arthrosc. May;18(5):638-43

6. Uquillas, C.A., Guss, M.S., Ryan, D.J., Jazrawi, L.M., and Strauss, E.J., 2015, Everything Achilles: Knowledge Update and Current Concepts in Management: AAOS Exhibit Selection. J Bone Joint Surg Am. Jul 15;97(14):1187-95

7. Pećina, M.M., Krmpotić-Nemanić, J., Markiewitz, A.D., (authors), 2001, Tunnel Syndromes. CRC Press; 3 edition August 16

8. Maigne, J.Y., and Maigne, R.; 1991, Trigger point of the posterior iliac crest: painful iliolumbar ligament insertion or cutaneous dorsal ramus pain? An anatomic study. Archives of Physical Medicine and Rehabilitation, 72(10):734-737]

9. Applegate, W.V., 2002, Abdominal Cutaneous Nerve Entrapment Syndrome (ACNES): A Commonly Overlooked Cause of Abdominal Pain. The Permanente Journal/ Summer Volume 6 No 3

10. Jacobs, D., 2011, What is the operator model? What is the interactor model? Self-published online

11. Jacobs, D.F., Silvernail, J.L., 2011, Therapist as operator or interactor? Moving beyond the technique. (letter) Journal of Manual and Manipulative Therapy Vol. 19 No. 2

12. Morrison, I., Löken, L.S., Minde, J., Wessberg, J., Perini, I., Nennesmo, I., and Olausson, H., 2011, Reduced C-afferent fibre density affects perceived pleasantness and empathy for touch. Mar 4; 134(4): 1116-1126

13. Øberg, G.K., Normann, B., and Gallagher, S., 2015, Embodied-enactive clinical reasoning in physical therapy. Physiother Theory Pract. May; 31(4):244-52

7. SOCIAL GROOMING – LESS IS MORE

"Monkeys, and other animals, groom each other often with a marked reduction in stress. Touch is good, and one doesn't need to wrap it up in pseudoscientific nonsense for it to be beneficial." - Mark Crislip MD, discussing reflexology on Science Based Medicine blog (Crislip 2010)

Manual therapy, maybe *all* health care (Benedetti 2010), probably evolved biologically as social grooming in primates and pre-language humans. All the neurobiological pathways, molecules, neurons, and synaptic proteins for appreciating social touch and physical care from another, are still all there in us (Haggard et al. 2013; Ryan and Grant 2009; de Wiljes et al. 2015; Olausson et al. 2002; Morrison et al. 2010).

This book has been about many ways we might, as manual therapists, affect the nervous system—all of it *at once*.

Consideration of a nervous system, according to me, includes considering the entire nervous system from skin cell (the part we can touch) to sense of self - the person, person's brain, spinal cord, and nerves, any physiological trouble that peripheral nerves might be in, any pain that may be present, any unconscious motor output that remains when a person is recumbent, and any volitional motor output that does not seem easy or effortless.

These are my assumptions and confirmation biases:

1. As a new patient walks in the door, I will only get a single chance to make a first impression.
2. The patient knows him or herself better than I ever will.
3. I am just a consultant they hire, a very privileged consultant with a license to touch people.
4. During the initial interview, the patient *and* their brain will be watching, listening, judging my ability to listen and reflect accurately, and help them sort their feelings and ideas.

5. I "know" I can touch skin, can plausibly deform the skin organ, and thus physically affect the nerves inside it (Lundborg 1988).

6. I "know" that nerves come all the way out to skin, that I can affect sensory input from there, and that there will only be three neurons between skin and processing areas of my patient's brain (Mason 2011).

7. Deforming the nerves in the skin organ of a person with an intact nervous system can send new input through neurons into their nervous system, into all its levels of operation, conscious or non-conscious.

8. Descending modulation of a favourable kind can be stimulated in the brain stem by more rostral centers; trust is a very big ingredient (Benedetti 2010). I also "know" I have no control over that.

9. I "know" that nocebo effect exists, that it creates cholecystokinin in the brain, which negates formation of endogenous opioids, and that I must try to think of everything I can to keep my environment, speech, demeanour free from it. (Benedetti 2010)

10. There are always going to be mountains I just cannot climb; some rare kinds of pain that I cannot help with, and people who will not feel comfortable around me for one reason or another; but I also feel pretty sure that the more years I have put into doing this work, the better I have become at doing it. (Hargrove 2015)

WHAT ABOUT US?

Given all this nebulousness and unknowableness and lack of certainty and the problems with studying manual therapy to develop an evidence base for it, should we even bother with trying to preserve manual therapy by reconceptualising it?

Does it matter what we think we're doing while we do it?

Yes! And yes!

Todd Hargrove (2015), one of the most succinct bloggers and writers on the topic of physical well-being, puts it well:

1. If you know how something works, you can make it work better:

   "... if my target was breaking up fascia or muscle knots then indeed I wouldn't care how [clients] felt. And I wouldn't do as good of a job."

2. Unintended consequences (of erroneous beliefs):

   "Misconceptions cost [clients] significant time, money, anxiety, and confusion."

   (I would add also, frustration, and often extra nociceptive input that no one should have to put up with, and which may simply sensitize the system more.)

3. The truth matters:

    "The truth has inherent value, even when its practical application is not immediately obvious. Knowledge is always powerful - for you, your clients, and the whole community."

    "As observers we are also creators building complementary pictures of inexhaustible reality. As agents our simplest behaviour will have repercussions, probably unsuspected, in many systems which concern us. And, above all, whether as observers or agents, we are ourselves part of the systems we seek to understand and to change or sustain." - G. Vickers (1981), quoted by Quintner et al. (2008).

    "Taking touch from physiotherapy is like asking a psychotherapist not to speak, or like taking the scalpel from a surgeon." ~ Chris Worsfold PT

LESS IS MORE

Examine your manual therapy assumptions, and confirmation biases, constantly.

Provide patients with favourable context:

1. Provide a comfortable treatment environment.
2. Listen. Listen. Listen. Your patient's brain will map *you, and how well you listen*, right into its own pathways, and the patient's own story.
3. Ask lots of questions to get more detail. Listen to the answers.
4. Provide plenty of pain education. Weave their own personal details into the new story you are now telling to them.
5. Explain what you intend to do, and why. Explain how the treatment is likely to feel. Make sure they understand they are in charge of the handling, and can interrupt it at the slightest discomfort. Ask permission to touch them before you touch them, even though it may seem perfectly obvious to both of you that physical contact is going to be part of the treatment contract.
6. Examine them thoroughly. Do not make any remarks that could potentially be noceboic.
7. Treat them slowly, thoughtfully, and carefully. Keep your hands clean, warm, slow, light, responsive, intelligent.
8. Above all, do no harm.

Be the best warm, helpful, engaged human with a skill set to offer that you can be. Be patient and use all your acute, well-honed listening skills, as best you possibly can.

"By our attitude to the other person we help to determine the scope and hue of his or her world; we make it large or small, bright or drab, rich or dull, threatening or secure. We help to shape his or her world not by theories and views but by our very attitude towards him or her. Herein lies the unarticulated and one might say anonymous demand that we take care of the life which trust has placed in our hands." — *Knud Løgstrup, Danish philosopher (quoted by Hintze et al. 2015)*

Recently I came across a set of principles called the "ethics of proximity" (Hintze *et al.* 2015), which I think beautifully describes the attitude we need to assume in order to create safe context for our patients:

1. When interacting with another, we have an ethical obligation to help the other.

2. What constitutes "helping" can be defined through discourse but must always respect the other's self-determination.

3. To interact authentically with the other is to risk ourselves and give up some of our control over where the dialogue between us takes us.

4. Do what works in the particular situation, taking from any other ethical field (especially discourse ethics, but also virtue, utility, or duty) but always respecting the other as the primary virtue.

5. In bringing preconceptions and prejudgments to our interaction with the other, we dismiss his needs.

6. When in a position of power over another, we are obliged to act in his best interest, not our own.

7. A relationship of caring has as its goal that of helping the other to gain his autonomy
   ~ From Table 4 Core Principles of Proximity Ethics, page 9, Hintze et al. 2015

I think all manual therapists should write these principles down on a piece of paper and tape them to the fridge, read them every day, embody them. If we adhere to these, we are already well on our way to helping people with manual care for pain problems.

REFERENCES

1. Crislip, M., 2010, Reflexology. Insert Nancy Sinatra Reference Here. Blogpost Science-Based Medicine Blog, Oct8. Retrieved May 12 2016. https://www.sciencebasedmedicine.org/reflexology-insert-nancy-sinatra-reference-here-2/

2. Benedetti, F., (Author), 2010, The Patient's Brain: The Neuroscience behind the doctor-patient relationship. Oxford University Press; 1 edition Nov. 14

3. Haggard, P., Iannetti, G.D., Longo, M.R., 2013, Spatial Sensory Organization and Body Representation in Pain Perception. REVIEW Volume 23, Issue 4, 18 February, Pages R164–R176

4. Ryan, T.J., and Grant, S.G.N., 2009, The origin and evolution of synapses. Nat Rev Neurosci. Oct;10(10):701-12.

5. de Wiljes, O.O., van Elburg, R.A.J., Biehl, M., and Keijzer, F.A., 2015, Modeling spontaneous activity across an excitable epithelium: Support for a coordination scenario of early neural evolution. Front Comput Neurosci. 9: 110

6. Olausson, H., Lamarre, Y., Backlund, H., Morin, C., Wallin, B.G., Starck, G., Ekholm, S., Strigo, I., Worsley, K., Vallbo, A.B., Bushnell, M.C., 2002, Unmyelinated tactile afferents signal touch and project to insular cortex. Nat Neurosci. Sept.; 5(9):900-4.

7. Morrison, I., Löken, L.S., Olausson, H., 2010, The skin as a social organ. Exp Brain Res. Jul; 204(3):305-14

8. Lundborg, G., 1988, Nerve Injury and Repair. New York. Churchill Livingstone

9. Mason, P., (Author), 2011 Medical Neurobiology. Oxford University Press, USA; 1 edition May 19.

10. Hargrove, T., 2015, Three reasons it matters why a treatment works. BetterMovement blog, Nov 5, retrieved May 12, 2016. http://www.bettermovement.org/blog/2015/three-reasons-it-matters-why-a-treatment-works

11. Vickers, G., (Author), 1981, Some implications of systems thinking. In: Open Systems Group, eds. Systems Behaviour, 3rd edition. London: Harper and Row, Publishers; 19–25. Quoted by Quintner et al, 2008

12. Quintner, J.L., Cohen, M.L., Buchanan, D., Katz, J.D., and Williamson, O.D., 2008, Pain Medicine and Its Models: Helping or Hindering? Pain Medicine Vol 9 No 7, 824–834

13. Worsfold, C., 2013, quoted by Chartered Society of Physiotherapy; Physio 13: Physiotherapy without touch is like psychotherapy without speech, conference told. Oct 16

14. Hintze, D., Romann-Aas, K.A., and Aas, H.K., 2015, Between You and Me: A Comparison of Proximity Ethics and Process Education. International Journal of Process Education. June, Volume 7 Issue 1

CPSIA information can be obtained
at www.ICGtesting.com
Printed in the USA
BVHW02s2234250318
511566BV00019B/185/P

9 781987 985184